In the final chapters of *Research Fraud in the Behavioral and Biomedical Sciences*, the editors explore, in great detail, options for future prevention of research fraud.

A comprehensive scholarly treatment of research fraud in the behavioral and biomedical sciences, this fascinating and enlightening book is essential reading for professionals in psychology, psychiatry, medicine, and related fields, and all those in the social sciences, as well as upper-level students in these disciplines.

About the editors

DAVID J. MILLER, PhD, is Coordinator of Automated Information Systems for the Department of Veterans Affairs, Mental Health and Behavioral Sciences Service, and Chair of the Bioethics Committee at the VAMC, Pittsburgh, Pennsylvania. An Assistant Professor of Psychiatry at the University of Pittsburgh School of Medicine, he is a former director of clinical training at the Pittsburgh VA Psychology Internship Consortium and Coordinator of the Center for the Evaluation and Treatment of Former Prisoners of War. Dr. Miller has published numerous papers in the areas of bioethics, posttraumatic stress disorder, and statistical modeling.

MICHEL HERSEN, PhD, is Professor of Psychiatry and Psychology at the University of Pittsburgh School of Medicine. Dr. Hersen also serves as the director of that university's postdoctoral training programs in psychiatry and in child psychiatry. He is a past president (1978–1980) of the Association for the Advancement of Behavior Therapy. Dr. Hersen's books include *Adult Psychopathology and Diagnosis* (coedited with S. M. Turner), *Handbook of Comparative Treatments for Adult Disorders* (coedited with A. S. Bellack), and *Treatment of Family Violence* (coedited with R. T. Ammerman).

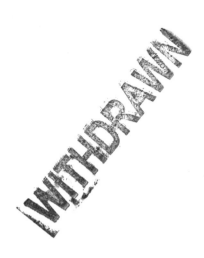

Research Fraud in the Behavioral

and Biomedical Sciences

RESEARCH FRAUD IN THE BEHAVIORAL AND BIOMEDICAL SCIENCES

Edited by

David J. Miller
Michel Hersen

John Wiley & Sons, Inc.

New York • Chichester • Brisbane • Toronto • Singapore

This publication is designed to provide accurate and
authoritative information in regard to the subject
matter covered. It is sold with the understanding that
the publisher is not engaged in rendering legal, accounting,
or other professional service. If legal advice or other
expert assistance is required, the services of a competent
professional person should be sought. *From a Declaration
of Principles jointly adopted by a Committee of the
American Bar Association and a Committee of Publishers.*

Library of Congress Cataloging-in-Publication Data

Research fraud in the behavioral and biomedical sciences / David J.
Miller and Michel Hersen, editors.
    p.   cm.
Include bibliographical references.
ISBN 0-471-52068-3 (alk. paper)
1. Research—Moral and ethical aspects. 2. Fraud in science.
3. Psychology—Research—Moral and ethical aspects. 4. Social
sciences—Research—Moral and ethical aspects. 5. Medical sciences—
Research—Moral and ethical aspects. I. Miller, David J., 1956–   .
II. Hersen, Michel.
    [DNLM: 1. Ethics, Professional. 2. Research—standards.
3. Scientific Misconduct. W 20.5 R428]
Q180.55.M67R47 1992
174'.2—dc20
DNLM/DLC   91-21625
for Library of Congress

Printed and bound in the United States of America by Braun-Brumfield, Inc.

10 9 8 7 6 5 4 3 2 1

To our wives, families, and colleagues,
who have exemplified the highest levels of integrity

Contributors

EUGENE BRAUNWALD, MD
Chairman, Department of
  Medicine
Hersey Professor of the
  Theory and Practice of
  Medicine
Brigham and Womens
  Hospital
Boston, Massachusetts

ROBERT P. CHARROW, JD
Crowell and Moring
Washington, DC

ALEXANDER J. CIOCCA, JD,
  MPH
Associate Legal Counsel
University of Pittsburgh
  Medical Center
Pittsburgh, Pennsylvania

RICHARD L. COHEN, MD
Professor Emeritus
Department of Psychiatry

University of Pittsburgh
  School of Medicine
Pittsburgh, Pennsylvania

THOMAS M. DILORENZO,
  PhD
Associate Professor and
  Chairman
Department of Psychology
University of Missouri–
  Columbia
110 McAlester Hall
Columbia, Missouri

DANIEL X. FREEDMAN, MD
Judson Braun Professor of
  Psychiatry and
  Pharmacology
Department of Psychiatry
  and Biobehavioral
  Sciences
School of Medicine
University of California
Los Angeles, California

MICHEL HERSEN, PHD
Professor of Psychiatry and
  Psychology
University of Pittsburgh
  School of Medicine
Department of Psychiatry
Western Pyschiatric
  Institute and Clinic
Pittsburgh, Pennsylvania

ARTHUR R. JENSEN, PHD
Professor of Educational
  Psychology
School of Education
University of California
Berkeley, California

DAVID J. MILLER, PHD
Program Coordinator,
  Automated Information
  Systems
Department of Veterans
  Affairs
Pittsburgh, Pennsylvania

ALAN POLING, PHD
Professor of Psychology
Department of Psychology

Western Michigan
  University
Kalamazoo, Michigan

MICHAEL J. SAKS, PHD,
  MSL
Professor of Law
College of Law
University of Iowa
Iowa City, Iowa

KENETH F. SCHAFFNER,
  MD, PHD
Professor of History and
  Philosophy of Science
  and
Adjunct Professor of
  Medicine
University of Pittsburgh
Pittsburgh, Pennsylvania

MARK H. THELEN, PHD
Professor of Psychology
Director of Clinical
  Training
Department of Psychology
University of Missouri–
  Columbia
Columbia, Missouri

Preface

Even as we are writing this preface, new cases of fraud and misconduct in the behavioral and biomedical sciences have been uncovered and are the subject of considerable attention and speculation. Indeed, the issue of fraud in research has received much media attention in the past several years, with journalists detailing the specifics of some spectacular cases. Unfortunately, these cases *may* represent only the tip of the iceberg; it is quite possible that such fraud in the behavioral and biomedical sciences is more widespread than is generally acknowledged.

Until recently, students in the medical, biological, and social sciences have been given only limited scholarly exposure to ethical issues in the research endeavor. This serious omission obviously needs to be rectified. We would hope that our book will fill the gap, given that our contributors have taken a meticulous and studied evaluation of the issues, at both the individual and instituitonal levels.

The book is divided into four parts, with Part I considering "General Issues." In the first chapter, the editors, Miller and Hersen, shed light on research fraud from a historical perspective, citing examples of scientific fraud and misconduct going back to antiquity. The point here is that fabrication of data and/or plagiarism is not new, but that the consequences in the 20th century have graver import. The second chapter, by Schaffner, considers empirical science from moral and ethical perspectives. The third chapter, by Charrow and Saks, considers the legal ramifications of fraud in science.

In Part II we evaluate "The Human Investigator Factor." Chapters 4, 5, and 6, respectively by Braunwalk, Miller, and Jensen, carefully examine histories of contemporary researchers alleged to have committed serious fraud and plagiarism. In Chapter 7 Miller looks at those personality factors that place the researcher at greater risk for committing the ultimate scientific misdeed. Finally, in Chapter 8, Poling details the unfortunate consequences of fraud.

Part III presents "System Considerations and Safeguards." In Chapter 9 Thelen and DiLorenzo consider the academic pressures influencing all researchers. Freedman (Chaper 10) examines the editorial process in relation to scientific fraud. Then, in Chapter 11, Cohen and Ciocca discuss the role of the institutional review board in providing ethical safeguards.

Part IV (Epilogue) contains Chapter 12, by Hersen and Miller, and suggests directions for the future. The emphasis here is on prevention at a systems level.

Many individuals have contributed graciously to the development and fruition of this project. First of all we thank our most erudite contributors, who agreed to share their thinking with us, albeit perhaps painful at times. We should acknowledge that we purposefully recruited individuals with strong and divergent opinions, with whom we do not always agree, because we thought their viewpoints needed to be formally articulated.

Second, we thank our support staff, Mary Newell and Mary Anne Frederick, for their technical assistance. Finally, we thank Herb Reich, our editor at John Wiley & Sons who agreed as to the timeliness of our book.

DAVID J. MILLER
MICHEL HERSEN

Pittsburgh, Pennsylvania
February 1992

Contents

Research Fraud in the Behavioral

and Biomedical Sciences

General Issues

Misconduct and Fraud in the Empirical Sciences: History and Overview

DAVID J. MILLER, PhD
MICHEL HERSEN, PhD

INTRODUCTION

As early as 1830, British mathematician Charles Babbage outlined his impression of researcher behavior that compromised the basic tenents of empirical investigations. Babbage outlined examples of scientific misconduct, which he referred to as "cooking" and "trimming" data to agree with a researcher's stated hypothesis. However, although he acknowledged fraud as a potential problem for science, he went on to state: "The cook [i.e., scientist] would procure a temporary reputation. . . at the expense of his permanent fame," and he implied that the actual occurrence of such misconduct was negligible (cited in Merton, 1957, p. 651). Perceptions about the perpetrators of fraud have not changed dramatically since Babbage's day. Such individuals are seen as "deviants," whose "tarnished reputations" must be brought to the attention of the general public. Subsequently, their writings are to be purged from the archival literature, with editors issuing statements of retraction.

In considering the incidence and prevalence of fraud and misconduct, there are widely varied perceptions of the true base rates. In a frequently cited editorial, Daniel Koshland (1987) of *Science* maintains that over 99% of scientific reports are "accurate and truthful," and in its booklet to nascent scientists, the National Academy of Science Committee on the Conduct of Science (1989) states that there is "good reason for believing the incidence of fraud in science to be quite low" (p. 15). Nevertheless, an analysis of routine audits conducted by the United States Food and Drug Administration from 1977 to 1988 shows that this low percentage is questionable. Indeed, data reveal that serious deficiencies were detected in 12% of the audits conducted prior to 1985. There is some optimism, however, because the rate appears to have diminished to 7% after 1985 (Shapiro & Charrow, 1989). But if the Shapiro and Charrow report that identifies serious problems with 7% of all FDA studies is generalizable to all research monies, a significant amount possibly is being expended on "questionable research."

It is not surprising, then, that the public may not view this smaller percentage as being an accurate reflection of scientific misconduct. The 1990 report by the Committee on Government Operations cites an 1989 AMA survey which reportedly found that 17% of the public believes research fraud happens "a lot" and an additional 41% believes it happens "a fair amount." Similarly, a survey of scientists found that 32% suspected a colleague of falsifying data and 32% suspected a colleague of plagiarism (Tangney, 1989). The U.S. government evidently had enough concern about problematic behavior within science to develop two agencies to scrutinize the scientific community. The Office of Scientific Review (OSR) is responsible for monitoring (or when warranted, conducting) investigations of scientific misconduct at Public Health Service grantee institutions. The Office of Scientific Integrity Review (OSIR) reviews results of such investigations and recommends sanctions to the Assistant Secretary of Health in the Department of Health and Human Services (Bivans, 1990. Although much anecdotal evidence exits, from an empirical perspective it is clear that research on base rates of scientific fraud and misconduct are lacking, and conclusions simply are at the speculative level.

Additional problems arise because of the varied definitions for fraud and/or misconduct. In Chapter 2, Schaffner outlines the differences between fraud (fabrication, fudging, and suppression of results) and other violations of professional norms that may be conceptualized as instances of misconduct (plagiarism and breaches of scientific etiquette). Levine (1988) defines fraud as the conscious and deliberate reporting in the scientific community of "facts" that the scientist knows are unsubstantiated. Such reporting is especially abhorrent if the investigator has "cooked" (i.e., fabricated) the data.

Since the days of Babbage there has been a dramatic shift in the criteria for an individual scientist's success, the scope of scientific inquiry, and the interaction between technology and science. Fraud and misconduct in the behavioral and biomedical sciences are of special concern because the conduct of the day-to-day operations of science (e.g., large laboratories and multisite collaborative investigations) and related economic considerations have changed considerably in the past 20 years. No longer are individual scientists and their endeavors monetarily supported through the private funds of the nobility (e.g., The Grand Duke of Tuscany's support for Galileo and Prince George of Denmark's support for Sir Isaac Newton). To the contrary, most research is supported through public funds (e.g., competitive grants) private monies (e.g., the various foundations or endowments), or private industry (e.g., pharmaceutical corporations). In the public sector alone, according to the 1990 report by the Committee on Government Operations, the U.S. government will spend approximately $21 billion for basic and applied research. The National Institutes of Health (NIH) research will receive more than $7 billion, and the Alcohol, Drug and Mental Health Administration, $763.7 million dollars. In an earlier era, personal prestige and professional recognition were the primary reasons to choose science as a career. Currently, however, in addition to those traditional factors for selecting a scientific career, universities and private industry offer individual researchers very potent monetary inducement.

PURE SCIENCE AND THE PURSUIT OF TRUTH

In his massive three-volume *Introduction to the History of Science*, George Sarton (1927) acknowledges that scientists are not necessarily more intelligent than artists, philosophers, or theologians. However, he does imply that knowledge gained through empirical means is more extensive and more accurate than beliefs acquired through other means. He argues: "The acquisition and systematization of positive knowledge [through science] is the only human activity which is truly cumulative and progressive" (p. 4). Sarton traces Western empirical science through the rediscovery of the body of Hellenistic knowledge (from the Muslim texts) combined with the pragmatic implications for technology of advanced Aristotelian logic, which essentially removed scientific thought from the body of faith (that was more closely akin to that of theology). Reflecting on this view, Lundberg (1947) stated: "When we [society] give our undivided faith to science, we shall possess a faith more worthy of allegiance than many we have vainly followed in the past, and we shall also accelerate the translation of our faith into actuality" (p. 144). This new hypothetico-deductive approach encouraged a pragmatic empiricism and was the forerunner of current scientific beliefs. Hence, the view of an objective, rational pursuit of a Platonic truth (which exists independently of the particular investigation and can be "discovered" through the proper combination of scientific procedure) dominated Western intellectual thinking throughout the 19th and early 20th centuries. It was assumed that scientists (i.e., those who attempted to discover the "truths") were part of a profession aware of and maintaining a shared set of values about the preeminence of the "empirical" nonbiased, conduct of scientific inquiry. All competent scientists presumably had an ideal mix of personality characteristics, including intelligence, perception, energy, productivity, insightfulness, synthetic ability, enthusiasm, oral expression, written expression, and analytic abilitities (Sindermann, 1982). At the same time, they were expected to be the repository of a large body of commonly held knowledge about the appropriate design, analysis, and reporting of empirical investigations. Finally, every scientist was supposed to hold a set of personal moral/ethical values that included veracity and an implied, but not usually articulated, awareness of his or her own personality characteristics that might lead to deviation from such ideals. Additionally, because scientists presumably held these values, individuals who chose science as a career were believed to be immune from the pressures of academic environments, financial inducements, or relative "power" considerations within academic/vocational environments. As late as 1957, sociologist Robert Merton stated:

> Like other social institutions, the institution of science has its characteristic values, norms, and organization. . . like other institutions, science has its system of allocating rewards for performance of roles. These rewards are largely honorific, since even today, when science is largely professionalized, the pursuit of science is culturally defined as being primarily a disinterested search for truth, and only secondarily, a means of earning a livelihood.

Science and scientists were seen as "pure," rational, and objective, and the responsibility for scientific fraud and misconduct was placed wholly on the individual researcher who perpetrated the offense. The belief was held that there was an inherent flaw in the personality structure, the familial upbringing, or a genetic weakness in that individual (Hilgartner, 1990). Implementation of this attitude into the actual day-to-day conduct of science is perhaps best exemplified through the writings of B. F. Skinner (1953):

> Science is first of all a set of attitudes. . . . It is characteristic of science that any lack of honesty quickly brings disaster. Consider, for example, a scientist who conducts research to test a theory for which he is already well known. The result may confirm his theory, contradict it, or leave it in doubt. In spite of any inclination to the contrary, he must report a contradiction just as readily as a confirmation. If he does not, someone else will—in a matter of weeks or months or at most a few years—and this will be more damaging to his prestige than if he himself had reported it. . . . In the long run, the issue is not so much of personal prestige as of effective procedure. Scientists have simply found that being honest—with oneself as much as with others—is essential to progress. Experiments do not always come out as one expects, but the facts must stand and the expectations fall. The subject matter, not the scientist, knows best. (p. 13)

Hence, individuals who choose a scientific career adopt an ethical position about the set of behaviors that we refer to as *scientific inquiry.* Behaviors are acceptable when they conform to a rule of conduct that meets the requirements of a supreme principle of duty (i.e., toward the pursuit of a Platonic, empirically derived truth). The moral rightness of an investigator's action does not consist in its being instrumental (directly or indirectly) to the realization of a good end, but in its being a kind of action that the moral law requires all scientists to perform as a matter of principle (Taylor, 1975). Scientists translated this combination of deontological, logical positivism into a faith based on rationalism and the empirical method: "All *definite* knowledge—so I should content—belongs to science; all *dogma* as to what surpasses definite knowledge belongs to theology" (Russell, 1945, p, xiii).

Science was seen as a "self-correcting" institution through its belief in the necessity of public verifiability and replication and took into account honest, human errors: The classic example was the case of the "N-rays." In 1903, approximately the same time that Roentgen discovered X-rays (1895) and Becquerel identified radioactivity (1896), Rene Blondlot, a French physicist, announced the discovery of what he termed the *N-ray* (named for Nancy University, his employer). Within 3 years hundreds of papers had been written about *N-rays*, and Blondlot was awarded the prestigious Prix Lecomte by the French Academy of Sciences. In 1904, however, Blondlot attempted to demonstrate the existence of N-rays for the visiting American physicist R. W. Wood. Unable to see the effect, Wood secretly removed part of the apparatus necessary to produce it. When the unknowing French continued to see the rays (even though their equipment was not working), Wood published his account rejecting the notion that N-rays even existed. It should be noted that at no time were the proponents of N-rays accused of fraud, in that no one charged them with consciously misrepresenting the results of their studies. In fact, it was Blondlot who had invited Wood to France (Burke, 1985). It was also true that the scientific community purged itself of this particular error in a relatively brief period.

There also were isolated reports of cases, that by contemporary standards, seem to have been clear instances of fraudulent behavior. For example, in 1912 British scientists Charles Dawson and Arthur Wooodword announced that they had found evidence of an apelike person in the gravel pits at Piltdown in southern England. Numerous unsuccessful attempts were made to relate their findings to hominids later discovered in Germany, China, South Africa, and Java. The final verdict was rendered in 1950 by Kenneth Oakley, who proved that the skull was that of a modern human, the jaw being from an ape, with the bones stained and the molars filed down. Particularly enigmatic is that the motivation for the Piltdown hoax remains unknown; the entire case was viewed as an anomaly and not indicative of potential problems within the scientific community.

THE REDEFINITION OF TRUTH

There may be, however, other reasons for fraudulent behavior and scientific misconduct. Lundberg (1929) stated that a scientist's "greed for applause" may become greater than his or her devotion to truth. It was believed that questionable behavior was essentially the result of scientific infighting that aimed at documenting the priority of a particular scientific discovery. Merton (1969) states: "The fact is that almost all of those firmly placed in the pantheon of science—Newton, Descartes, Leibnitz, Pascal, or Huyghens, Lister, Faraday, Laplace, or Davey—were caught up in passionate efforts to achieve priority and to have it publicly registered" (p.7). Sir Isaac Newton is perhaps the prototype of a brilliant scientist who may be accused, not of altering the data he collected, but of participating in less than honorable conduct in establishing his place in history. Specifically, when the German mathematician Leibnitz appealed to the Royal Society to assess relative claims, between him and Newton, for the discovery of calculus, the President of the Society (Sir Isaac) appointed a committee consisting of his adherents, directed the committee's activities, and anonymously wrote the preface for the published report (Merton, 1969; Hawking, 1988). Additionally, Newton had battles with Robert Hooke, a mathematician, calling him alternatively a "fool" and a "charlatan," and finally accusing him of pirating ideas from others (Merton, 1957). But despite Newton's questionable practices, the community of fellow researchers held that his *science* nonetheless was correct, his *data* pure, and his *conclusions* about scientific propositions valid.

Beginning in the 1960s there was a perceptible shift in the conceptualization of philosphers and historians of science with respect to the purity of the research endeavor. Out of the earlier existential questioning of "reality," "linearity," "progression," and "meaning," Thomas Kuhn (1970) in his historic work, *The Structure of Scientific Revolution*, explores the process of scientific knowledge and inquiry. Briefly, Kuhn's thesis purports that knowledge gained through scientific inquiry is not always the result of the rational, objective, civilized discourse of unbiased researchers. What is held as conventional knowledge by a particular group of scientists will be tested and shaped into what Kuhn refers to as a *normal science*. Hence, scientists will accumulate data that substantiate a commonly held belief although it may not necessarily be the most accurate explanation of a particular phenomenon. A period of normal sicence may last for decades, even centuries, and will develop a unique language, historians, and defenders of its "truths." Eventually, and inevitably, when the anomalies of a particular belief system outweigh that which is explained, a revolution occurs, along with the eventual paradigm shift to another period of normal science. Oft-cited examples include the radical shift in scientific beliefs from pre- to post-Copernican, Darwinian, and Einsteinian thinking.

There are numerous examples of the exclusion of alternative explanations by normal science. For example, in 1769, "thunderstones" (i.e., meteors) were submitted from several independent sources to the French Academy of Sciences. However, because the evidence was collected by "common persons" (rather than "scientists"), the Academy did not consider evidence that could explain the origin of meteors. Only after the French Revolution (and the concomitant rise of status for the commoner) was the scientific community convinced of the potential usefulness of data collected by persons not schooled in the art of science. Additionally, in 1915, the German meteorologist, Alfred Wegener published his theory of what we now refer to as *continental drift*. His ideas were rejected by British and American scientists even though he had geological evidence to support his claim. Unfortunately, he died as an intellectual outcast. Currently, astronomer Halton Arp (1990) accuses the field's leadership of restricting his admittedly unorthodox inquiries. Arp (1990), who bases his work on renegade Nobel prize winner physicist Hannes Alfven, complains that he is unable to obtain necessary time on telescopes necessary to perform his experiments because "the strong personalities in the field. . . feel it necessary that *they* decide what is right and wrong for everyone else" (Marshall, 1990, p. 15).

Proponents of the nonlinear view of scientific progression argue that the eventual acceptance of a given paradigm over another is as much a function of such nonrational factors as the individual personalities of proponents of one belief system or a set of historical/cultural factors. Karl Popper (1985) states:

> What we should do, I suggest, is to give up the idea of ultimate sources of knowledge, and admit that all human knowledge is human: that it is mixed with our errors, and our prejudices, our dreams, and our hopes: that all we can do is to grope for truth even though it is beyond our reach. We may admit that our groping is often inspired, but we must guard against the belief, however deeply felt, that our inspiration carries any authority, divine or otherwise. (p. 57)

Popper's view may account for an explanation of how alleged phenomena, such as N-rays, were accepted by legitimate and rational scientific persons for so long a period of time (Blondlot believed in their existence until his death in 1930). One potential explanation is centered on the state of the French- German political situation in the early 1900s. Apparently the French scientific community was feeling particularly threatened by its German counterpart and in need of a new discovery to bolster its reputation. Broad and Wade (1982) quote historian Mary J. Nye in stating that the proposal of N-rays was not the result of irrationality, a pseudoscience, or psychopathology on the part of Blondlot. It was, however, probably the consequence of "the structure of Blondlot's scientific community, its organization, aims and aspirations around 1900" (p. 114).

Recently, Kuhn's conceptualizations have been criticized and revised (Lakatos & Musgrave, 1970; see also Chapter 2 in this volume). Briefly, the modifications acknowledge that whether science is construed as more or less a collection of solutions to puzzles, we currently possess greater knowledge about those puzzles and are able to exert more control over our environment and physical health than in the past. It may be that, as Kuhn would suggest, all we know is more about the answers to a shared set of assumptions constituting our idiosyncratic view of "reality," but at least we do know more of those answers. The major value of a Kuhnian analysis here lies in its emphasizing on *process* of science (nonlinear as it may be) and in assisting the empirical sciences to more adequately pursue their lofty goals.

LEVELS OF RESPONSIBILITY

In an incisive evaluation of fraud and misconduct in science, Hilgartner (1990) presents a tripartite analysis of the division of responsibility with regard to misconduct in science. The first level, is the *causal* analysis, which examines *institutional factors*. That is, the day of the independent and solo investigator has been over for some time. In fact, even in the 17th century, Isaac Newton gathered what we now might view as a "think tank" of mathematicians and astronomers. Currently, large-scale, multisite collaborative investigations pose their own set of potential difficulties, including data sharing, coauthorship, and possible breaches of confidentiality. Furthermore, the Association of Academic Health Centers recently (1990) published a report examining potential conflicts of interest in university-based medical centers. Finally, much attention has been given to the interaction between the development and sale of applied technology by academicians and academic institutions (Patent Rights and Technology Transfer, 1990; Levine, 1990). Misconduct and fraud in this context have been attributed to numerous factors, including the "publish or perish" pressure; a "grant or get going" mentality of major grant-driven institutions; lack of mentorship; and inadequate replication, record keeping, and storing of old data. These are discussed in greater detail in Part III of this volume.

The second level is the moral analysis, which considers the unique role of the individual in perpetrating fraud or misconduct. Part II of this book explores case examples in detail. For example, most recently, charges of misconduct have been alleged in the so-called *Cold Fusion* incident. Briefly, in 1989 researchers Stanley Pons and Martin Fleischman, from the University of Utah, gained immediate fame by claiming that a room-temperature, test-tube nuclear reaction could produce enough heat to be a viable source of commercial power. In disseminating their results Pons and Fleishman presented their data to the public media rather than through the more traditional peer-reviewed channels. As a consequence, many of their colleagues expressed outrage that the investigators had initiated a "media blitz" (Pool, 1990; Pool, 1991).

The debate over cold fusion continues with two recently published books. Physicist Frank Close (1991) alleges that Pons and Fleishman committed a "serious error in judgment" in their representation of experimental results, maintaining that the original claim was so "skewed as to be invented" (Broad, 1991, p. 1). However, MIT science writer Eugene Mallove (1991) believes that physicists have administered a coup de grace to a promising field of inquiry and have overlooked an auspicious field of inquiry (Hamilton, 1991a, p. 1415).

Another complicated example of fraud involves the case of Theresa Imanishi-Kari who, it appears, fabricated data during the course of her work in genetics (Hamilton, 1991b). From 1986 to 1989, investigative panels at MIT, Tufts, and NIH found "no evidence of fraud, manipulation, or misrepresentation of data." However, utilizing the forensic expertise of the U.S. Secret Service, a congressional inquiry by Representative John Dingell cast doubt on those conclusions. Specifically, when compared with other data tapes made at the same laboratory, those presented by Imanishi-Kari were allegedly created at a different time (Anderson, 1990a; Anderson, 1990b). Unfortunately, the case had been further complicated because one of her co-authors and continued supporters was Nobel Prize winner and President of Rockefeller University: David Baltimore (Weaver et al., 1986; Fackelmann, 1990). However, as of March 21, 1991, Dr. Baltimore reversed his position, stating that his coauthor made assertions as to the veracity of experiments without evidence to support them (Baltimore, 1991). In addition, an NIH panel found that Imanishi-Kari "fabricated key data" (NIH: Imanishi-Kari guilty, 1991, p. 262). (See Part II of this book for a more comprehensive analysis of the issues involved in specific cases.)

The *third* level of analysis involves *political considerations*, including the activities of the agencies and their personnel responsible for rectifying the problems of fraud and misconduct in science. Hilgartner (1990) also identifies four strategies that possibly can be carried out to limit the occurrence of scientific fraud and misconduct in the future: (1) a "law enforcement" strategy of detection, deterrence, and punishment; (2) an "oversight" policy emphasizing data and quality assurance monitors; (3) an "educational" approach that oversees preventive efforts; and (4) a system that reinforces scientific integrity rather than mere productivity.

AIM OF THIS BOOK

In the succeeding chapters our aim is to present a scholarly examination of the issues. Our eminent contributors will (1) elucidate various problems in the current scientific system, (2) provide guidelines to researchers and institutions for preventing such occurrences, and (3) recommend to administrators and governmental officials policy development that will enable them to monitor more effectively the huge behavioral and biomedical research enterprise.

REFERENCES

Anderson, C. (1990a). New evidence emerges in Tufts misconduct case. *Nature, 347,* 317.

Anderson, C. (1990b). Science meets forensic science. *Nature, 347,* 507.

Arp, H. (1990). Discordant observations. *Science, 249,* 611.

Association of Academic Health Centers. (1990). *Conflicts of interest in academic health centers* (Policy Paper #1). Washington, DC: Author.

Baltimore, D. (1991). Dr. Baltimore says "sorry." *Nature, 351,* 94–95.

Bivans, L. (1990). Scientific records and regulations. *Science, 248,* 1471.

Broad, W. J. (1991, March 17). Cold Fusion claim is faulted on ethics as well as science. *The New York Times,* pp. 1, 30.

Broad, W., & Wade, N. (1982). *Betrayers of the truth.* New York: Touchstone.

Burke, J. (1985). *The day the universe changed.* Boston: Little, Brown and Company.

Close, F. (1991). *Too hot to handle: The race for cold fusion.* Princeton: Princeton University Press.

Committee on Government Operations. (1990). *Are scientific misconduct and conflicts of interest hazardous to our health?* (Report No. 19). Washington, DC: U.S. Government Printing Office.

Fackelmann, K. A. (1990). Secret Service questions data authenticity. *Science News, 137,* 310.

Hamilton, D. P. (1991a, March 22). Cold fusion: Battle of the books. *Science, 251,* 1415.

Hamilton, D. P. (1991b). Verdict in sight in the "Baltimore Case." *Science*, *251*, 1168–1172.

Hawking, S. W. (1988). *A brief history of time*. Toronto: Bantam.

Hilgartner, S. (1990). Research fraud, misconduct, and the IRB. *IRB: A review of human subjects research*, *12* 1–4.

Koshland, D. E. (1987). Fraud in science. *Science*, *235*, 141.

Kuhn, T. S. (1970). *The structure of scientific revolutions* (2nd ed., enlarged). Chicago: University of Chicago Press.

Lakatos, I., & Musgrave, A. (1970). *Criticism and the growth of knowledge*. Cambridge, England: Cambridge University Press.

Levine, J. (1990). Technology tales. *Johns Hopkins Magazine*. Baltimore: Author.

Levine, R. J. (1988). *Ethics and regulation of clinical research* (2nd ed.). New Haven, Yale University Press.

Lundberg, G. A. (1929). *Social research*. New York: Longmans Green.

Lundberg, G. A. (1947). *Can science save us?* New York: Longmans, Green, and Co., Inc.

Mallove, E. (1991). *Fire from ice: Searching for truth beyond the cold fusion furor*, New York: Wiley.

Marshall, E. (1990). Science beyond the pale. *Science*, *249*, 14–16.

Merton, R. K. (1957). Priorities in scientific discovery: A chapter in the sociology of science. *American Sociological Review*, *22*, 635–651.

Merton, R. K. (1969). Behavior patterns of scientists. *American Scientist*, *57*, 1–23.

National Academy of Science. (1989). *On being a scientist*. Washington, DC: National Academy Press.

NIH: Imanishi-Kari guilty. (1991). *Science*, *350*, 262–263.

Patients Rights and Technology Transfer. (1990). The University of Pittsburgh (Document #11-02-01). Pittsburgh, PA: Author

Pool, R. (1990). Cold fusion: Only the grim remains. *Science*, *250*, 754–755.

Pool, R. (1991). High noon in Utah. *Science*, *251*, 371.

Popper, K. R. (1985). *Popper selections*. Princeton, NJ: Princeton University Press.

Russell, B. (1945). *A history of western philosophy*. New York: Simon & Schuster.

Sarton, G. (1927). *Introduction to the history of science*. Baltimore: Williams & Wilkins.

Shapiro, M. F., & Charrow, R. P. (1989). The role of data audits in detecting scientific misconduct: Results of the FDA program. *Journal of the American Medical Association*, *261*, 2505–2511.

Skinner, B. F. (1953). *Science and human behavior*. New York: The Free Press.

Sindermann, C. J. (1982). *Winning the games scientists play*. New York: Plenum Press.

Tangney, J. P. (1987). Fraud will out—or will it? *New Scientist, 115*, 62–63.

Taylor, P. W. (1975). *Principles of ethics: An introduction*. Belmont, CA: Wadsworth.

Weaver, D., Reis, M. H., Albanese, C., Constantini, F., Baltimore, D., & Imanishi-Kari, T. (1986). Altered repertoire of endogenous immunoglobin gene expression in transgenic mice containing a rearranged Mu Heavy chain gene. *Cell, 45*, 247.

Ethics and the Nature of Empirical Science

KENNETH F. SCHAFFNER, MD, PhD

INTRODUCTION

A number of authors have characterized science, and in particular the natural sciences, as "value-free."[1] Although this thesis is defensible in a narrow sense, a more accurate picture of science will display values of two types that function centrally in all scientific disciplines. These two types can be termed *cognitive* and *social*; more will be said about them in the following section. In addition, a complete description of the scientific enterprise requires an account of what happens when these values are violated. One purpose of this

[1]See Rescher (1965) for comments on the widespread acceptance of the value-free nature of science, and a criticism of that thesis. For an analysis of the value-free character of the social sciences, and references to social scientists who argued for such a position, including Max Weber, see Nagel (1961), pp. 485–502.

volume is to provide several detailed case studies of an extreme but important violation of scientific norms: scientific fraud.

The concept of *scientific fraud* can be defined as intention[2] to deceive the scientific community about the nature of scientific results, whether these be empirical or theoretical (cf. the National Academy of Science analysis by its Committee on the Conduct of Science, Ayala et al. 1989, p. 9068). Fraud in science is viewed as a spectrum of behaviors, with three principal subtypes: (1) fabrication (or "forging"), (2) fudging, and (3) suppression of results (typically data) (Zuckerman, 1977, p. 113; Ayala et al. 1989, p. 9068). In addition to fraud, the most grievous of professional crimes, it is also necessary to consider other breaches of professional norms to provide a complete picture of scientific values. These additional transgressions include plagiarism and other forms of scientific larceny, as well as suppression of scientific advances (Ben-David, 1977), and finally breaches of "scientific etiquette," such as self-eponymization (e.g., naming a scientific law after oneself) or the underacknowledgment of scientific collaborators' contributions (Zuckerman, 1977). In this book, in addition to a number of studies of scientific fraud, the problem of plagiarism is considered in the case of Dr. Alsabti (see Chapter 5).

The extent of scientific misconduct, including scientific fraud, is difficult to determine. Merton in 1942 alluded to "the virtual absence of fraud in the annals of science" (1942/1973), but in 1982 noted that quantitative data on the incidence of fraud were not available, and Kohn states that adequate data were still unavailable as of the writing of his book (1986, p. 7). A number of widely publicized cases are discussed in the present book, and others can be found in Broad and Wade (1982) and in Kohn (1986).

This chapter will first discuss the nature of scientific research and indicate how both cognitive and social values or norms are intimately intertwined with the structure of science. I will then discuss why violations of the norms represent serious problems for science and society and embed this discussion in the context of an ethical frame-

[2]The notion of *intentional* deception is a critical aspect of the nature of scientific fraud. Scientists can commit other errors that deceive either themselves or others *un*intentionally. See Ayala et al. (1989), pp. 9061–9064 and 9068–9069, for examples of scientific error and its relation to issues of fraud.

work that will assist professionals in making recommendations for alleviating these problems.

THE STRUCTURE OF SCIENCE AND THE NATURE OF SCIENTIFIC RESEARCH

Several decades ago it would have been unnecessary to preface a discussion about scientific fraud with an analysis of whether there *is* any "objective truth" in science. During the past 25 or so years, however, serious questions have been raised about the nature of scientific truth and progress by the influential work of Kuhn (1962/1970), as well as by some philosophers of science (e.g., Feyerabend, 1975) and several sociologists of science (Latour & Woolgar, 1979); a brief discussion of these issues may be helpful.

Truth and Progress in Science

Throughout this century, philosophers of science have engaged in vigorous disputes about the nature of scientific truth. An examination of the history of science in general and the biomedical sciences in particular would lead to the conclusion that many "good" scientific theories have not survived to the present day. Kuhn's (1970) characterization of scientific revolutions provides a superb (if ultimately misleading) introduction to examples of these discarded theories. Such theories have gone through the stages of discovery, development, acceptance, rejection, and extinction. Further examination of extinct theories, however, would show that they provided a number of valuable consequences for science. Incorrect and literally falsified theories have several explanatory functions, and have also systematized data, stimulated further inquiry, and led to other important practical benefits. For example, the false Ptolemaic theory of astronomy was extraordinarily useful in predicting celestial phenomena and served as the basis for oceanic navigation for hundreds of years. Newtonian mechanics and gravitational theory, which are incorrect from an Einsteinian and quantum mechanical perspective, similarly

served both to make the world intelligible and to guide its indus-
trialization. In the biological sciences Lamarck's false evolutionary
theory systematized and explained significant amounts of species
data, and in medicine Pasteur's false nutrient depletion theory of the
immune response nontheless served as the background for the development of the anthrax vaccine (Bibel, 1988, pp. 159–161). Such
examples lead toward what has been termed an *instrumentalistic*
analysis of scientific theories (or hypotheses). The basic idea behind
such a position is to view theories and hypotheses as tools and not as
purportedly true descriptions of the world. For a thoroughgoing instrumentalist, the primary function of scientific generalizations is to
systematize known data, to predict new observational phenomena,
and to stimulate further experimental inquiry. Such an approach bears
strong analogies to the "constructivist" program of several sociologists of science, such as Latour and Woolgar (1979), who conceive
many biomedical entities (e.g., neuroendocrine-releasing factors) as
being "constructed" rather than "discovered."

Although such a position is prima facie attractive, it is inconsistent
with other facets of scientific inquiry. For example, scientists view the
distinction between what they term *direct* and *indirect* evidence as
important. Even though (as I have argued elsewhere; Schaffner, in
press) the distinction is relative, it is nonetheless significant that
scientists *behave* as if the distinction is important, and that "direct
evidence" would seem to support a more *realistic* analysis of scientific theories (or hypotheses). A realistic alternative to the instrumentalist position would characterize scientific theories as *candidates*
for true descriptions of the world. Although not denying the importance of theories' more instrumentalistic functions, such as prediction
and fertility, the realist views these features as partial indications of a
theory's truth. The history of recent philosophy of science has seen an
oscillation between these realist and instrumentalist positions, as well
as the development of some interesting variants of these positions, a
subject that cannot be pursued within the limitations of this chapter
(but see Leplin, 1984, for a collection of recent articles in this area).

In spite of the varying positions that scientists and philosophers of
science have taken about the nature of ultimate scientific truth, they
do not disagree about the need for scientists to report accurately and
faithfully what they have observed or concluded in their investiga-

tions.[3] The seriousness of scientific fraud becomes understandable with the realization that perpetrating such fraud undermines the very nature of the scientific enterprise. Zuckerman (1977) quotes Medawar on this point:

> Scientists try to make sense of the world by devising hypotheses. . . . In the course of events scientists very often guess wrong, take a wrong view, or devise hypotheses that later turn out to be untenable. . . . Nor does [this] necessarily impede the growth of science because where they guess wrong, others may yet guess right. But they won't guess right if the factual evidence that led to formulating the hypothesis and testing its correspondence with reality is not literally true. For this reason any kind of falsification or fiddling with professedly factual results is rightly regarded as an unforgivable professional crime. (Medawar, 1976, p. 6)[4]

Cognitive Values in Science

Sociologists of science, beginning with the classical work of Robert K. Merton (1942/1973), have identified a number of norms or values. Generally these are distinguished into two classes: (1) cognitive (or technical) norms, including methodological canons; and (2) "moral" (or social) norms which prescribe (and proscribe) the reporting and crediting of the results of scientific investigations (see Merton, 1942/1973; Mulkay, 1969; NAS, 1989; Zuckerman, 1977). Cognitive norms encompass various principles of experimental design, the statistical analysis of evidence, and valid inferences from evidence, as well as more vaguely defined criteria for assessing scientific theories.

[3]An interesting side-issue raised by claims of scientists (such as Medawar, in his 1963 article, or Hanson, in his 1958 monograph) is whether scientists typically report the full process of their discoveries *as they actually happened*. These authors argue that the typical scientific article is a re-presentation of a scientist's work for the purposes of validation and reconfirmation. Although this is almost certainly the case, such re-presentation does not constitute fraud but is rather compliance with standard scientific practice.

[4]As a first approximation Medawar's statement is correct, but in the light of recent discussions about realism in philosophy of science, needs to be fine-tuned to ameliorate the force of terms such as *wrong*, *correspondence with reality*, and *literally true*. For references to the literature and a discussion of one form of such fine-tuning, see Schaffner (in press, Chapter 5).

There has been extensive discussion in the philosophy of science literature about the nature and the roles of such criteria, including experimental fit and "simplicity" (see Popper, 1959; Kuhn, 1970, esp. his postscript; Schaffner, 1970; Newton-Smith; 1981) that cannot be pursued here. It has been difficult to characterize in any succinct and temporally-universal sense what constitutes science and scientific methodology, a conundrum sometimes termed the *demarcation problem* (Popper, 1959; also see Ayala et al., 1989). Some philosophers have gone so far as to deny existence of a scientific methodology (Feyerabend, 1975), whereas others see the issue as requiring an appreciation of historically evolving principles (Shapere, 1984).

Moral (or Social) Scientific Norms

Most relevant for this chapter are the moral or social norms of science. In his pioneering (1942/1973) study, Merton proposed four such norms:

Universalism. This norm is similar to the cognitive norms in that it emphasizes the importance of objective or, in Merton's terms, "preestablished impersonal criteria," but it goes beyond the cognitive by explicitly disavowing any appeal to the scientist's "race, nationality, religion, class, and personal qualities. . . ." in scientific advances (p. 270)[5]

Communism (or communality)[6] This term refers to the belief that the "substantive findings of science are the product of social collaboration and are assigned to the community. . . [as] a common heritage. . . ." (p. 273). The existence of eponyms, patents, or copyrights does not falsify this belief, although patents may produce certain tensions in science (p. 275).

[5]It should be remembered that Merton's original publication of these norms occurred during the period of Nazi domination in Europe. Nazi ideology emphasized the validity of "race" in science, thus Merton's views had a heightened significance at that time.
[6]*Communality* is Barber's (1952) term, and it is better suited for describing the property introduced by Merton in his (1942/1973) essay.

Disinterestedness. This norm refers to a "distinctive pattern of *institutional* control" (my emphasis) of scientists' motives. Although Merton's discussion has somewhat unclear aspects, his description of this norm indicates that scientists will be motivated to search for scientific *truth*, in the sense of objective knowledge, and will not either be biased toward "pet" hypotheses or fraudulently offer evidence in support of such hypotheses, which if accepted, would (illicitly) advance their careers.[7] In connection with this norm Merton also refers to the "rigorous policing" that occurs in science through the verification of results. Merton believes that implementation of "disinterestedness" is the reason there is "virtual absence of fraud in the annals of science. . . ." (p. 276).

Organized skepticism. This norm requires subjecting a scientific claim to "the detached scrutiny of beliefs in terms of empirical and logical criteria" (p.277). As such, this norm appears to reemphasize an amalgam of the cognitive norms discussed earlier with disinterestedness."

Other writers have suggested additional moral norms or have proposed somewhat different terminology for Merton's original statements. Barber (1952) recommended individualism, rationality, and emotional neutrality, and Cournand and Zuckerman (1970) proposed honesty, objectivity, tolerance, doubt of certitude, and unselfish engagement (also see Zuckermann, 1977). Kohn (1986) also cites Mohr (1979), who proposes the following principles: "Be honest; never manipulate data; be precise; be fair with regard to priority; be without bias with regard to data and ideas of your rival; do not make compromises in trying to solve a problem."

It is the violation of these moral (or social) norms of science that constitutes the primary subject of this book.

---

[7]Kohn in his book (1986, p. 2) characterizes this value as follows: "Disinterestedness requires that the scientist's activities and efforts be directed toward the extension of scientific knowledge, and not towards the personal interests of an individual or a group of scientists."

THE NATURE OF ETHICS

Normative and Descriptive Ethics

The study of ethics can be approached from two somewhat different perspectives. Ethics can be studied from a *descriptive* point of view, in which the intent is to describe how individuals and groups behave and, perhaps, what these individuals or groups believe about the moral nature of their behavior. This approach is common in the social sciences, such as anthropology, and is typified by such statements as "the ancient Aztecs believed that human sacrifices in religious contexts were appropriate." Alternatively, ethics can be approached from a *normative* perspective, in which the investigator is attempting to determine *what* the ethically correct decision is in a set of circumstances, and *why* that is the case. Frequently the two approaches are mixed in the same essay, as in several of the articles cited earlier from the sociology of science. In the remainder of this chapter, I am going to be taking the *normative* perspective.

THE SUMMERLIN AFFAIR

The incidents associated with the research of Dr. William T. Summerlin exhibit several features of scientific fraud in a specific way. The Summerlin affair also provides a typical example of how institutions deal with the disclosure of such violations of scientific research values.

Dr. Summerlin, a dermatologist who had been conducting research on skin grafts since the late 1960s, moved to the Sloan-Kettering Cancer Institute in 1973 (Hixson, 1976; NAS, 1989, p. 9068). A protégé of Dr. Robert Good, the then recently named Director of the Institute, Summerlin's research was highly publicized as a breakthrough in immunology with important implications for cancer research. Summerlin claimed to have transplanted tissue between animals of different genetic strains, eliminating the transplant rejection barriers by growing the transplant in a laboratory nutrient broth culture. Summerlin's work involved skin grafts between mice and two genetic strains, the black C57 and the white A strains, as well as corneal transplants from humans to rabbits. In spite of a number of other laboratories' attempts to replicate Summerlin's positive results, confirmation was not forthcoming. In addition, one of Summerlin's own postdoctoral fellows was about to publish an article reporting the inability to verify his supervisor's well-publicized claims.

Summerlin was asked to present evidence of his research to Dr. Good, and after selecting specimens showing grey skin on a white mouse, Summerlin intentionally darkened the transplanted skin to make it appear as a black patch on a white strain. He offered this forged example of his work to Dr. Good, who accepted the results as prima facie evidence of Summerlin's claims. Several hours afterward, however, a laboratory technician noted that the mouse had been artificially darkened and that the ink was removable with alcohol. The technician reported this finding to Summerlin's fellow, who took the information to Dr. Good. Summerlin was immediately suspended, and a five-person peer-review committee was appointed by the Institute to examine Summerlin's research projects.

The committee reviewed the inked mouse example as well as Summerlin's research on transplanted corneas and concluded that "some actions of Dr. Summerlin over a considerable period of time were not those of a responsible scientist." The committee found no evidence that Summerlin had been able to outflank the immune rejection response in his skin graft experiments and further criticized his corneal transplant experiments as being incorrectly carried out and presented in a "grossly misleading" manner (Hixson, 1976, pp. 200–201). Summerlin was dismissed from the Institute for this behavior.

Principle-Based Normative Ethics

One approach to ethics might be termed "principle-based." This means that problems generated by cases such as the Summerlin affair are examined from the perspective of both current "rules" (or guidelines or policies) for dealing with those problems and several ethical principles to be defined later in this article. These principles are by design quite general. Acceptance of them entails prima facie duties (i.e., duties that may be overridden by other principles in the set, in the light of further ethical deliberations). The scientist, by referring both cases and rules to these principles and examining possible solutions to the problems in the light of whichever general ethical theory he or she holds, attempts to reach a specific recommendation that fits under a (possibly modified) rule. (The nature and role of general ethical theory will be discussed more fully later in this chapter.)

It is important to stress that there is no significant difference in form between moral reasoning and scientific reasoning as regards the need to think critically, to analyze various factors, and to synthesize possible solutions to problems, even though the content is different.

Some codes of scientific or medical ethics appeal only to guidelines

for action or to professional rules. Two examples from medical ethics
are "Maintain confidentiality," and "Always obtain informed consent." Scientific research ethics also has its rules, and some were
cited earlier from Mohr's (1979) work, for example, "Never manipulate data." These rules are not necessarily shown to be derived from
more general concepts when they are presented. Often such rules
come into conflict with one another when applied to an individual
case, and there may be no obvious reason to judge one as more
binding than another in that situation. Such rules, however, are actually statements for scientists about how to embody more general
ethical principles in their professional behavior. The principles themselves, then, may provide a more rational platform from which to
adjudicate conflicts.

The principles that can be employed will vary from writer to writer
(see Bok, 1977, for a discussion related to medical ethics and its
principles), but interestingly there is a surprising agreement in the
inner content of the ethical principles of most authors writing in ethics
generally, in research ethics, and in medical ethics. In the section on
moral (or social) norms I discussed some of these principles under the
rubric of *values* and *norms*. In the well-developed area of medical
ethics a small set of basic values was introduced in the *Belmont
Report* (*National Commission*, 1978) and was further developed and
applied by Beauchamp and Childress in their influential book
(1979/1983/1989) and in the many volumes produced by the President's Commission for the Study of Ethical Problems in Medicine and
Biomedical and Behavioral Research (1983). Because Beauchamp and
Childress's book is perhaps more systematic, general, and accessible
than these other publications, and because the publications of the
President's Commission for the Study of Ethical Problems in Medicine and Biomedical and Behavioral Research are perhaps the most
influential, I shall refer to both of their approaches to illustrate a
principle-based ethics.

Beauchamp and Childress begin from a position that resembles
Ross's (1930) system of prima facie duties. Ross, who falls into the
"deontologist" category of ethicist (see the discussion of ethical theory in the following section), argued that there were a number of
directly *intuited* fundamental ethical principles or values including
fidelity, reparation, gratitude, justice, beneficence, self-improvement,
and nonmaleficence (Munson, 1983; see pp. 21–26 for a good elemen-
tary discussion of Ross's views). Beauchamp and Childress proceed

from a similar position and define four ethical principles that they argue should be helpful in making ethical decisions. The President's Commission presents three basic principles or values, amalgamating two of Beauchamp and Childress's principles into one. These principles are:

> *Autonomy.* A person is autonomous if and only if he or she is self-governing; sometimes this principle is called *self-determination* (in particular, the President's Commission volumes presume that there is a basic "right to self-determination"). The individual then can legislate norms of conduct and is able voluntarily to fix a course of action. For an individual to acknowledge the ethical importance of the principle of autonomy for another is the basis for the closely related principle of *respect for persons.*
>
> *Well-being.* This principle has two major manestations:
>
> 1. *Nonmaleficence.* This (sub)principle has a Hippocratic basis and means "do no harm." This usually means both the prevention of harm and the removal of harmful conditions.
> 2. *Beneficence.* This (sub)principle refers to a duty to confer benefits or to help others further their important and legitimate interests.
>
> *Justice.* This principle refers to giving each person his or her "right to due." An individual is just toward another person if he or she gives that person what the person deserves or is owed. This notion is further developed in a set of "material principles of justice" such as "to each an equal share" or "to each according to merit."

As I noted earlier, these values are general tools used to clarify and extend rules and help to solve ethical problems in connection with specific cases. The values, in turn, are themselves justified, and conflicts among them are resolved by appeal to a still higher level, general ethical theory.

General Ethical Theory

Any discussion of general moral theory of necessity gets somewhat abstract; I do not, in this chapter, wish to elaborate on the topic in any depth but merely wish to state that there are two general types of ethical theory. One is based on evaluating the *consequences* of either individual acts or of rules in the light of some general goal, such as happiness or pleasure. The "consequentialist" theory has an influential subtype called *utilitarianism*, in which the individual should act to maximize the greatest happiness for the greatest number of people. Another quite different ethical theory is based on a general set of rules that are presumed to be right in themselves *regardless of the consequences*. This type of theory is called *deontological* and is associated historically with Kant, but presently with the Harvard philosopher Rawls (even though Rawls does permit taking certain consequences into account). Rawls's (1971) approach has also been termed *contractarian*. Another form of this theory that is quite influential in biomedical ethics is Ross's theory of prima facie duties expressed as a series of principles. These theories can help in moral deliberations by providing general perspectives from which to test decisions. The two types of theories are idealized "pure" types and most people borrow from both in reaching their decisions. This is not necessarily inconsistent, and some further comments on the nature of moral reasoning will make this point clearer.

Thus far I have introduced a number of general concepts such as values, rights, and utilitarian moral theory, as well as some specific examples such as "respect for persons" and "beneficence." Because of the complexities of the issues in this area of research ethics, it may be useful to elaborate how to go about resolving some of the moral dilemmas that arise in connection with such decisions.

Moral theories are intended to provide a general point of view for analyzing ethical problems and reaching a well-grounded decision. Arriving at such an ethical theory involves a usually lengthy and complex process of moral reasoning in which the individual works from a stock of given ethical principles as well as specific test cases. Rawls articulated this process well in his remarkable book, *A Theory of Justice* (1971), where he develops a method for reaching the state of reflective equilibrium. There he works back and forth between specific cases and general propositions, but many other ethicists have found it more useful to include several levels of moral appeal between cases and general ethical theories. I have found it useful in summarizing the preceding views and in thinking through the relations of various levels of ethical problem solving to use a modification of the process proposed by Beauchamp and Childress (1989). The following diagram is a convenient way to picture the interactions just described.

4. Ethical theories
↑ ↓
3. Ethical principles
↑ ↓
2. Rules or guidelines
↑ ↓
1. Particular judgments and actions in cases

It is possible to interpolate institutional policies as well as legal rules and principles into the preceding framework. This can be done through a review of the relevant policy documents governing an institution and also through a concurrent analysis of recent court decisions in relevant cases, aided by consultation with appropriate legal counsel. It is important, however, to avoid confusing institutional codes and/or legal principles with ethical principles, thereby reducing moral reasoning to policy/legal analysis.

In spite of the place of general ethical theories at the apex of the diagram, my approach places emphasis for problem solving at the level of principles. This view is close to that of the American philosophers Dewey and Tufts (1936), who wrote:

> [M]oral principles are the final methods used in judging suggested courses of action. . . . Their object is to supply standpoints and methods which will enable the individual to make for himself an analysis of the elements of good and evil in the particular situation in which he finds himself. . . .
>
> A moral principle, then, is not a command to act or forbear acting in a given way: it is a tool for analyzing a special situation, the right or wrong being determined by the situation, the right or wrong being determined by the situation in its entirety, and not by the rule as such. (p. 309)

APPLICATIONS AND IMPLICATIONS

From what has been stated thus far, it appears that a reasonably well-characterized group of values and rules govern scientific research. These values and rules are *normative* and represent an unofficial honor code for research scientists. Violation of these principles clearly calls for an institutional and perhaps a broader societal response, with appropriate sanctions imposed on those violating the principles. The Summerlin case is an instance of such deviant behavior,[8] and there are, unfortunately, many other infractions of scientific norms (see Part III for examples).

Confronting the code of research ethics with cases of research fraud and plagiarism provokes interesting questions, such as how widespread is such behavior and what steps should be taken to eliminate or control such behavior? Other chapters in this volume address these questions in detail (although, as noted earlier, firm quantitative data are hard to come by) and discuss possible remedies for solving such problems. In addition, the recent National Academy of Sciences report (Ayala et al., 1989) makes a number of recommendations in this area and also indicates that Sigma Xi, the American Association for the Advancement of Science, and other scientific and engineering organizations "are prepared to advise scientists who encounter cases of possible misconduct" (NAS, 1989, Ayala et al. p, 9072). The United States Congress continues to hold hearings into problems of research fraud, and the National Institutes of Health are in the process of developing guidelines for dealing with these problems. Such laws and guidelines as may be passed and issued will function at the second level in the schema presented in the preceding diagram, and it will fall to individuals and peer review committees that deal with instances of scientific conduct to apply those rules in the light of the ethical principles discussed earlier in this chapter.

Without additional data supporting a thesis of widespread fraud, it is difficult to agree with Broad and Wade's proposition (1982) suggesting that something is seriously wrong with the conventional ideology of science—essentially the picture I provided in the section "The Structure of Science and the Nature of Scientific Research." Broad and Wade cite historical episodes of purported fraud and misrepresentation, but they do so in a somewhat biased manner, and alternative interpretations are available (see Zuckerman, 1977). It is impor-

[8]The word *deviant* is the technical sociological term for behavior that lay persons refer to by "criminal" and "immoral" descriptors. See Zuckerman (1977) for examples of this approach and also references to the area.

tant to recognize the pressures and temptations that the current mileau of scientific practice can generate, however, and to counter such factors with appropriate educational materials. Some of these issues are discussed in the Ayala et al.'s NAS Report (1989), as well as in later chapters of this book. Additional information and analysis of data on scientific misconduct are needed, and they will likely be forthcoming from future sociological analyses of scientific practice.

SUMMARY

This chapter introduces definitions of types of scientific fraud and discusses such behavior in the context of the nature of empirical science, scientific research, and scientific norms. A brief analysis of whether there is any objective truth in science and the nature of the cognitive values of science is followed by an account of moral (or social) scientific norms. This account, which largely follows Merton and later sociologists of science, indicates why scientific fraud is rightly regarded as an unforgivable professional crime. An extended example—the Summerlin affair—illustrates this type of fraud. The chapter then discusses normative ethics, summarizes the currently favored "principle" orientation of biomedical ethics, and briefly examines ethical theory. The place of rules and guidelines in the hierarchy of normative ethics is indicated, and the last part of this chapter considers how scientists might begin to implement the ethical perspective outlined herein. It also provides several pointers to the literature and to institutional assistance available in this area.

REFERENCES

Ayala, F., Adams, R. M., Chilton, M.-D., Holton, G., Hull, D., Patel, K., Press, F., Ruse, M., & Sharp, P. (1989). On being a scientist. *Proceedings of the National Academy of Sciences USA, 86*, 9053–9074. (Also issued as an independently published booklet by the National Academy of Sciences)

Barber, B. (1952). *Science and the social order.* New York: Free Press.

Beauchamp, T., & Childress, J. (1989). *Principles of biomedical ethics* (3rd ed.). New York: Oxford University Press. (Earlier editions appeared in 1979 and 1983)

Ben-David, J. (1977). Organization, social control, and cognitive changes in science. In J. Ben-David & T. Clark (Eds.), *Culture and its creators: Essays in honor of Edward Shils* (pp. 244–265). Chicago: University of Chicago Press.

Bibel, D. J. (Eds.). (1988). *Milestones in immunology: A historical exploration.* Madison, WI: Science Tech.

Bok, S. (1977). The tools of bioethics. In S. J. Reiser, A. J. Dyck, & W. J. Curran (Eds.), *Ethics in medicine* (pp. 137–141). Cambridge: MIT Press.

Broad, W., & Wade, N. (1982). *Betrayers of the truth.* New York: Simon and Schuster.

Cournand, A., & Zuckerman, H. (1970). The code of science. *Studium Generale, 23,* 941–962.

Dewey, J., & Tufts, J. H. (1936). *Ethics* (revised ed.). New York: Henry Holt.

Feyerabend, P. K. (1975). *Against method.* London: New Left Books.

Hanson, N. R. (1958). *Patterns of discovery.* Cambridge: Cambridge University Press.

Hixson, J. (1976). *The patchwork mouse.* Garden City, NY: Anchor Press/Doubleday. (Appendix 1 contains the full text of the Report of Summerlin Peer Review Committee (May 17, 1974); Appendix 2 contains Dr. Summerlin's Statement of May 28, 1974, about the incident.)

Kohn, A. (1986). *False prophets.* Oxford: Basil Blackwell.

Kuhn, T. S. (1970). *The structure of scientific revolutions* (2nd ed.). Chicago: University of Chicago Press. (Originally published 1962)

Latour, B., and Woolgar, S. (1979). *Laboratory life.* Beverly Hills, CA: Sage.

Leplin, J. (Ed.). (1984). *Scientific realism.* Berkeley: University of California Press.

Medawar, P. (1963). Is the scientific paper a fraud? *The Listener 70:* 377–378.

Medawar, P. (1976). The strange case of the spotted mice. *New York Review of Books, 23,* 6–11.

Merton, R. K. (1973). The normative structure of science. In N. Storer (Ed.), *The sociology of science: Theoretical and empirical investigations* (pp. 267–278). Chicago: University of Chicago Press. (Originally published as "Science and Technology in a Democratic Order," *Journal of Legal and Political Sociology 1* (1942):115–126)

Mohr, M. (1979). The ethics of science. *Interdisciplinary Science Reviews, 4,* 45–53.

Mulkay, M. (1969). Some aspects of cultural growth in the natural sciences. *Social Research, 36,* 22–53.

Munson, R. (1983). *Intervention and reflection: Basic issues in medical ethics* (2nd ed.). Belmont, CA: Wadsworth.

Nagel, E. (1961). *The structure of science.* New York: Harcourt, Brace & World.

National Commission for the Protection of Human Subjects of Biomedical and Behavioral Research. (1978). *The Belmont Report: Ethical principles and guidelines for the protection of human subjects of research* (2 Vols.). Washington, DC: DHEW publication No. (OS) 78-0012.

Newton-Smith, W. (1981). *The rationality of science.* Boston: Routledge, Keegan Paul.

Popper, K. R. (1959). *The logic of scientific discovery.* New York: Free Press.

President's Commission for the Study of Ethical Problems in Medicine and Biomedical and Behavioral Research. (1983). *Summing up.* Washington, DC: U.S. Government Printing Office. (This volume is a general review of the Commission's publications; see Appendix D for a complete list of publications and their tables of contents.)

Rawls, J. (1971). *A theory of justice.* Cambridge: Harvard University Press.

Rescher, N. (1965). The ethical dimension of scientific research. In R. G. Colodny (Ed.), *University of Pittsburgh series in philosophy of science: 2. Beyond the edge of certainty* (pp. 261–276). Englewood-Cliffs, NJ: Prentice-Hall.

Ross, W. D. (1930). *The right and the good.* Oxford: Clarendon Press.

Schaffner, K. F. (1970). Outlines of a logic of comparative theory evaluation with special attention to pre- and post-relativistic electrodynamics. In R. Stuewer (Ed.), *Minnesota studies in the philosophy of science* (Vol. 5, pp. 311–364). Minneapolis: University of Minnesota Press.

Schaffner, K. F. (in press). *Discovery and explanation in biology and medicine.* Chicago: University of Chicago Press.

Shapere, D. (1984). *Reasons and the search for knowledge.* Dordrecht: Reidel.

Zuckerman, H. (1977). Deviant behavior and social control in science. In E. Sagarin (Ed.), *Deviance and social change* (pp. 87–138). Beverly Hills, CA: Sage Publications.

Legal Responses to Allegations of Scientific Misconduct

ROBERT P. CHARROW, JD
MICHAEL J. SAKS, PhD, MSL

INTRODUCTION

This is a tale of two agencies and their efforts to deal with the issue of scientific misconduct. It is a saga rife with internal political intrigue, acrimonious congressional hearings, and deep-seated disagreement over the government's role in regulating the integrity of science (Broad & Wade, 1982; Olswang & Lee, 1984; O'Reilly, 1990; Van de Kamp & Cummings, 1987; Woolf, 1988). Above all, the story has a moral: It is impossible to avoid legal entanglements by ignoring legal formalities.

One agency, the Food and Drug Administration (FDA), confronted the problem directly, using well-established and carefully articulated legal norms. As a result, during the past decade it has swiftly and effectively resolved numerous cases of alleged scientific misconduct without embarrassing publicity or debilitating federal court litigation (Shapiro & Charrow, 1985, 1989).[1] In contrast, the other agency, the National Institutes of Health (NIH), despite congressional pressure, resisted efforts to reform its procedures for resolving cases of misconduct. Rather than employing the adversarial procedures used by the FDA, the NIH opted to resolve cases of misconduct through an informal process known as the scientific dialogue paradigm. It attempted to transmute a highly charged, inherently adversarial process into an even-tempered collegial debate. In so doing, it sacrificed focus, formality, and the types of procedural protections normally expected when peoples' reputations are at stake. Moreover, it sowed seeds of discontent that only now are beginning to blossom in the federal courts. In short, this is a story of science, politics, and the law and how a science-funding agency can misuse the law to thwart political pressures.

ACT 1: THE EMERGING PROBLEM

Scene 1: The National Institutes of Health

In the late 1970s and early 1980s, the number of reported cases of scientific misconduct increased dramatically; almost all of them involved biomedical research. Stimulated by a series of cases that came to light in 1980, the Subcommittee on Investigations and Oversight (chaired by Rep. Albert Gore (D-TN)) of the Committee on Science and Technology convened hearings in April 1981 (1) to ascertain whether the reported cases were anomalies or instead the tip of the iceberg, and (2) to determine whether universities and federal funding

---

[1]The FDA, unlike other federal agencies, does not have an explicit definition of scientific misconduct. Researchers who undertake grossly deficient research are subject to disciplinary action whether or not their conduct was intentional. The Public Health Service, NIH's parent agency, defines misconduct in science as "Fabrication, flasification, plagiarism, or other practices that seriously deviate from those that are commonly accepted within the scientific community for proposing, conducting, or reporting research. It does not include honest error or honest differences in interpretations or judgments of data." 54 Fed. Reg. 32,446, 32,449 (August 8, 1989), codified at 42 C.F.R. § 50.102.

agencies were doing an adequate job of detecting and resolving cases of misconduct (Woolf, 1988). During these hearings, the research community argued that scientific misconduct was such a rare phenomenon, at most an aberration, that intrusive prophylactic procedures were unwarranted. Thus, government regulation to ensure the integrity of science not only was unnecessary but also would set an ominous precedent. Based on such representations, the subcommittee took no action.

By 1985, however, the Congress lost patience. Responding to new evidence that the procedures used by universities and the NIH for handling cases of misconduct were ad hoc, less than prompt, and frequently inadequate, the Congress enacted section 493 of the Public Health Service Act, codified at 42 U.S.C. § 289b.[2]

Section 493 required the Secretary of Health and Human Services to issue rules requiring, among other things, that awardee institutions establish "an administrative process to review reports of scientific fraud," and "report to the Secretary any investigation of alleged scientific fraud which appears substantial." The law also required the Director of the NIH to create a process for promptly responding to information provided by awardee institutions.

In short, the Public Health Service Act, as amended, placed the primary responsibility for investigating and resolving allegations of misconduct on the awardee institutions. In that regard the law was unique. For the first time, a nongovernmental entity was required to investigate allegations of improper conduct by its employees and to turn that information over to the federal government. Defense contractors are under no similar obligation. The law, however, was not self-executing, and the Congress left it to the Secretary to issue implementing regulations.

Soon thereafter the NIH amended its *Guide for Grants and Contracts* (NIH, 1986) to include the procedures that it would use and that grantees should use in resolving cases of misconduct. (See the section "Policies and Procedures for Dealing with Possible Misconduct in Science.") Unfortunately, the new provisions did little more than memorialize the ad hoc process that the NIH had been using for years. The NIH continued to adhere to the notion, attacked by Congress,

[2]See H. R. Rep. No. 99-309, 99th Cong., 1st Sess. 83-84, accompanying the Health Research Extension Act of 1985, Pub. L. 99-158.

that cases of misconduct are best handled informally, scientist-to-scientist, outside the normal administrative process. Specifically, provisions of the *Guide* set out a two-stage process. Upon receiving a complaint, an awardee institution was to institute a preliminary review of the evidence to determine whether it warranted a more formal investigation, the university was to apprise the NIH once a formal investigation had started, and was to inform the NIH of the results of that investigation when it ended.

The NIH reserved the right to undertake an investigation of its own if it believed that the university's investigation either was not proceeding apace or was inadequate. The *Guide* did not define the procedures by which the NIH would make determinations of misconduct, but it did set out the sanctions that the Department could impose without a formal administrative hearing (see NIH *Guide*, pp. 21–23).

Shortly after the *Guide* was published, the NIH announced the adoption of its ALERT system. Once an accused is under investigation his or her name is entered into the ALERT computer system, which apprises NIH personnel of a pending action by either an awardee institution or the NIH against an investigator. This information could be used by the NIH in deciding whether to award a pending grant or whether to appoint an individual to an advisory committee.[3]

The NIH hoped that these interim measures would placate both the Congress and those in the Department of Health and Human Services who believed that a more coherent, efficient, and formal process was needed.

Scene 2: The Federal Food and Drug Administration

In sharp contrast, during this same period, the Food and Drug Administration, the NIH's sister agency within the Public Health Service, developed and implemented an aggressive and well-defined system for detecting and resolving cases of misconduct. Although the FDA does not fund research, it relies on the results of clinical drug trials in assessing whether to approve a new drug for marketing. Under the provisions of the Federal Food, Drug, and Cosmetic Act, as amended, a manufacturer of a new drug must demonstrate both its safety and efficacy before marketing the drug. Initially, a manufac-

[3]See 52 Fed. Reg. 19,929 (May 28, 1987).

turer must file a notice of claimed investigational exemption for a new drug. This permits a physician, under contract with the manufacturer, to administer the investigational new drug to human subjects following a specific protocol.

During the mid-1970s, the FDA, in part stimulated by the wave of published reports of misconduct in science, became concerned with the integrity of data it received as part of the drug approval process (see Olswang & Lee, 1984; O'Reilly, 1990; Van de Kamp & Cummings, 1987). Accordingly, in 1977 it established an office to conduct on-site data audits. The FDA used two types of audits. Routine data audits were conducted of studies that might form the basis for drug approval or that are otherwise judged to be important (Kelsey, 1978). In addition, the FDA may be prompted to conduct for cause audits of some investigators who have not been subjected to routine audits if someone, usually a colleague or an employee, informs the FDA that something might be amiss, or if the FDA receives a complaint about the clinician from a drug manufacturer or harbors suspicions about the validity of an investigator's data.

The audit function was coupled with a prosecutorial function and a set of well-delineated procedures that could end with a ruling by the Commissioner disqualifying the investigator from receiving investigational new drugs.[4] Specifically, if an audit suggested that an investigator had engaged in scientific misconduct, he or she would be so advised and given an opportunity to respond. If the response proved inadequate, the FDA would then advise the individual of its intent to disqualify him or her from doing future clinical trials. At that point, the accused could request a formal trial-like hearing under the provisions of the Administrative Procedure Act (APA). At the hearing, an FDA attorney would act as a prosecutor and both that attorney and the accused's attorney would have the opportunity to call, confront, and cross-examine witnesses.

The FDA program has been a success in a number of respects. First, researchers who have conducted fraudulent or grossly negligent research have been detected and weeded out of the system. For instance, between 1977 and 1989, 47 formal disqualifications were made, 26 by consent settlements. Second, the process is relatively

[4]21 C.F.R. Part 312 (1990).

expeditious compared with NIH standards. And third, no one has challenged its legality.

Clearly the types of problematic research reviewed by the FDA can be, and frequently are, qualitatively different from the research that would be under scrutiny by NIH investigators. The FDA data are clinical, thereby permitting the agency to check the validity of the data by reviewing patient records or by interviewing the patients themselves. In contrast, NIH-funded research frequently involves highly specialized in vitro experimentation that may well be at the cutting edge of science. Ascertaining the validity of that type of research is far more difficult for several reasons. First, although a generalist may be able to review and understand clinical records, such is frequently not the case with the types of research that the NIH funds. Only those with experience in the specialty involved are in a position to evaluate the authenticity and merit of the work. Even then, the avenues for verifying suspect data are limited. The data can be checked for internal consistency and against laboratory records, or those who ostensibly witnessed the experiments being performed (or not being performed) may be able to provide direct evidence as to what occurred. In short, the NIH's task is likely to be far more complex than the FDA's.

Moreover, the reader should not infer that the FDA's surveillance program, which involves on-site data audit of significant clinical trials, is either feasible or desirable for NIH-funded research. Quite to the contrary, a data audit program would be ill-advised and impractical for a variety of reasons. First, the FDA has a legitimate interest in verifying the accuracy of clinical data. After all, it must rely on those data to carry out its responsibility of deciding whether to approve a new drug for marketing. The NIH, on the other hand, is not a regulatory agency. The data generated by grantees are not directly used to shape or otherwise influence public policy. Second, a data audit program in the basic sciences might well represent an inappropriate intrusion into the practice of science. And third, such a program would place an unwarranted premium on record keeping and conformity. Although this may be a laudable and necessary goal in clinical drug trials, it may well have adverse effects on basic researchers. It could stifle creativity and chill the free and open interchange of information and ideas that is so essential in the growth of scientific knowledge.

In short, although the FDA's audit program may be inappropriate for NIH-funded research, the procedures that it uses for resolving cases of misconduct in clinical trials may be entirely appropriate.

ACT II: THE PROBLEM SWALLOWS THE SOLUTION

While the FDA was busy implementing and refining its procedures for dealing with misconduct, the NIH should have been busy developing rules to implement the mandate set forth in Section 493. For the next 3 years, the Department and the White House sporadically wrestled with the problem of how best to implement the provisions of the Extension Act. The matter, though, was not high on anyone's agenda.

Events, however, would soon overtake the Department. While the DHHS was studying the issue, weighing alternatives, and debating linguistic nuances, the Congress was conducting hearings, criticizing funding agencies, and hinting that it would adopt sweeping remedial legislation. The congressional hearings conducted by two subcommittees in 1988–1989 were particularly significant because of their focus and what they portended (House Committee on Energy and Commerce, Subcommittee on Oversight and Investigations, 1988; House Committee on Energy and Commerce, Subcommittee on Oversight and Investigations, 1989; House Committee on Government Operations, Human Resources, and Intergovernmental Relations Subcommittee, 1988). Although the hearings were ostensibly aimed at assessing the ability of the NIH to deal with allegations of misconduct, the staffs of the various subcommittees attempted in certain instances to judge the merit of some research. This culminated in the highly publicized set of hearings conducted by Congressman John Dingell's subcommittee into allegations that the NIH, Tufts University, and the Massachusetts Institute of Technology mishandled their respective investigations into charges that an article coauthored by Nobel Laureate David Baltimore contained data allegedly falsified by Baltimore's coauthor Theresa Imanishi-Kari.

Following the Baltimore hearings, many in the research community learned that Dingell and other interested House members were drafting sweeping legislation to ensure the morality of scientists. The legislation was viewed by many as draconian. In an effort to thwart this legislative effort, the DHHS quickly published a notice of proposed rulemaking (NPRM) codifying some of the NIH's interim policies and procedures for dealing with cases of misconduct.[5]

Among other things, the proposed rule would require universities receiving NIH funding to adopt procedures, consistent with due process, for resolving allegations of misconduct. Although the rules would leave universities free to fashion their own procedures, they codified the two-step process, originally set out in the *Guide*, that universities were required to use. First, upon receiving a complaint or other information, the university would be required to institute an inquiry to determine whether there was reason to believe that scientific misconduct had occurred. If it had, the institution would then have to undertake a more formal investigation and report that fact to the NIH. The NPRM also established time lines for the inquiry and investigation and further required that the final report following the investigation be submitted to the NIH.

As the comment period to the NPRM was drawing to a close, concern was growing within the Department that Congress would take preemptive action by enacting legislation that (1) would further regulate the entire area of misconduct, and (2) would transfer some of the NIH's jurisdiction to the HHS Office of Inspector General. To address these concerns, the DHHS, through its Task Force on Scientific Misconduct, considered a number of proposals to reorganize the Department's oversight responsibilities. One proposal recommended that the investigative and monitoring functions previously undertaken by the NIH be transferred to a new office outside that agency, and further, that an adjudicative process, akin to the one used by the FDA, be employed. A competing proposal, championed by the Public Health Service, sought to maintain the status quo but to increase resources available to the NIH for dealing with misconduct.

In the end, the Department adopted a compromise solution by creating two new offices.[6] The first, the Office of Scientific Integrity (OSI), would be part of the NIH and would be responsible for monitoring investigations conducted by universities, undertaking investigations of its own where it believed that a university had failed to do an adequate job, and instituting inquiries and investigations into

[5]53 Fed. Reg. 36,347 (Sept. 19, 1988).
[6]54 Fed. Reg. 11,080 (March 16, 1989).

allegations of misconduct lodged against intramural scientists at the NIH and the Alcohol, Drug Abuse and Mental Health Administration. The second office, known as the Office of Scientific Integrity Review (OSIR), would be part of the Office of the Assistant Secretary for Health. The OSIR, among other things, would review investigations conducted by the OSI and recommend appropriate sanctions to the assistant secretary. In short, the HHS sought to address the problem of misconduct in science in the best tradition of government—by creating more government.

The seeds of discontent that eventually would culminate in federal court litigation were sown with the creation of OSI and OSIR. Both offices were established in response to political exigencies. Neither office had a clear charge. To complicate matters, the Department's misconduct rules, which became final in August 1989, were aimed entirely outward at the universities.[7] There were no duly published rules governing OSI and OSIR. Consequently, although the HHS requires universities to have written policies for dealing with allegations of misconduct, it never published in the *Federal Register*, as required by law, the procedures that it would use in conducting investigations. Instead, OSI continued to adhere to the belief that its investigations were best conducted in an informal, nonadversarial environment with the rules for each case being tailored to the needs of that case.

Although the tenor and scope of OSI investigations might vary from case-to-case, all investigations were conducted using the so-called "scientific dialogue" process. Under that process, OSI investigators would interview witnesses, review laboratory notebooks, make findings of fact, and propose recommended sanctions, where appropriate, all without the benefit of a formal trial-like hearing. In short, the accused was not offered, and in the NIH's view not entitled to, the same protections that the Department generally accorded others accused of serious legal infractions.

Thus, as the decade of the 1980s came to a close, the NIH had made relatively little progress in grappling with the issue of scientific misconduct. Although it grudgingly admitted that there might be a problem, it attempted to thwart congressional criticism by reorganizing offices, reassigning personnel, and increasing resources. The NIH,

[7] 54 Fed. Reg. 32,446 (Aug. 8, 1989).

though, never addressed the underlying problems with its procedures. The rule that it published in 1989 did little more than codify the informal set of procedures orginally published in 1986. Those procedures failed adequately to address the early congressional concerns— they were still informal, ad hoc, and inefficient. These deficiencies would soon lead to litigation.

ACT III: NIH GOES TO COURT

In 1990 two cases, under the aegis of the NIH, found their way into the ederal courts. One case, initiated by a research scientist under investigation by OSI, involved a direct challenge to the legality of OSI procedures. The other case, instituted by a disgruntled whistle-blower against a researcher and his employing universities, sought monetary damages in the form of a federally sanctioned reward under the *qui tam* provisions of the False Claims Act. Both posed serious challenges to the system that the NIH had been using for resolving cases of alleged misconduct.

Scene 1: The Abbs Affair

In July 1990, James Abbs, a tenured professor of neurology and neurophysiology at the University of Wisconsin at Madison, instituted suit against the NIH seeking to enjoin OSI from undertaking an investigation into allegations that Abbs had engaged in scientific misconduct (*Abbs and The Board of Regents of the University of Wisconsin v. Sullivan*, 1990). The complaint alleged, among other things, that OSI procedures denied Abbs due process under the Fifth Amendment and were, therefore, constitutionally infirm. The case is instructive for a variety of reasons. First, it evidences the scientific community's growing frustration with OSI. Second, the record in the case dramatizes what can best be described as an egregiously slow process. And third, it underscores the shaky legal basis of OSI operations.

The case began typically enough on April 7, 1987, when Steven Barlow, a former graduate student of Abbs, wrote a letter to the journal *Neurology* accusing Abbs of altering or falsifying data in an article that he had published in that journal. Barlow claimed that a graph Abbs had published in the article had been modified from a graph that Abbs and Barlow had published in a 1983 article appearing in the *Journal of Speech Impaired Research* (*sic*).[8] Barlow sent copies of his letter to the University of Wisconsin and to the NIH, which had funded Abbs's reseach.

Soon thereafter, the University, through a committee, conducted an initial inquiry into Barlow's charges and in the following month unanimously concluded that Barlow's allegations were "unsubstantiated and [did] not justify or require a more formal investigation" (see Plaintiff's Joint Proposed Findings of Fact and Conclusions of Law in *Abbs v. Sullivan* at § 61 (August 20, 1990)). The University forwarded those conclusions to the NIH's Office of Extramural Affairs.

The University had resolved the matter in approximately 1 month; the NIH took considerably longer. Court documents indicate that the Abbs inquiry was under episodic review within the NIH for almost 3 years. Abbs contended that the NIH had in fact reviewed the University's findings and judged them to be satisfactory. The NIH, however, contended that it had never reached a definitive conclusion. Instead, it asserted that "two internal NIH committees reviewed the materials and failed to reach a definitive conclusion" (Statement, 1990, p. 3). In either event, the NIH's interest in the case was rekindled when, in 1988, the agency was contacted by an unidentified scientist who had been following the Abbs affair in the scientific press. The scientist suggested that for a variety of statistical reasons Abbs' position was not tenable.

In January 1990, Abbs was formally notified that he was the subject of an OSI investigation and that his name had been placed into the ALERT system. On June 4, 1990, a visiting team from the OSI sought to interview Abbs. As a precondition to the interview, however, Abbs' attorney sought assurances from OSI's legal counsel that Abbs would be afforded an opportunity to review the evidence gathered by OSI, and further that he would have the right to call and cross-examine witnesses. The OSI refused to give these assurances and

---

[8]Although we give the journal name as it appears in the Transcript of a Special Scientific Panel in re: University of Wisconsin, 3 (June 4, 1990) we do not believe any periodical by this name does (or should) exist. At any rate, we cannot find one by this name.

noted that there would be no trial-like hearing unless the Department decided to seek the most severe sanction—governmentwide debarment.

Shortly thereafter, Abbs instituted his suit. The following month the University of Wisconsin joined Abbs as another party plaintiff. The University's involvement ultimately would prove crucial to the disposition of the case. Whereas Abbs relied primarily on lofty principles of due process, the University concentrated on a considerably more arcane issue: whether the OSI procedures were void under the Administrative Procedure Act (APA).[9]

The parties received a taste of things to come during an oral argument on the plaintiffs' motion for a preliminary injunction. The federal judge hearing the case opined from the bench that she was "shocked"[10] by the OSI procedures, that those procedures "were the work of amateurs,"[11] and that "it would be embarrassing. . . to defend them."[12] Nonetheless, she stated that "unless Dr. Abbs can show that he's about to lose his job—and as you point out he has tenure at the University, that's not a probability—it's unlikely that he can succeed on the merits of his challenge to these procedures."[13] Before ruling, she asked the parties to submit briefs on the various legal issues.

On December 31, 1990, the court upheld the constitutionality of OSI's procedures, but simultaneously invalidated those procedures on technical grounds of the Administrative Procedure Act.

Under the APA, an agency is precluded from issuing final rules that may affect segments of the general public unless it has first gone through notice-and-comment rulemaking which is designed to permit the public to comment on agency proposals. Normally, a proposed rule is first published in the *Federal Register*; the public is then given an opportunity to file comments about the proposal with the agency. Those comments are reviewed by agency personnel, appropriate changes are made in the proposal, and the final rule is then published. The hallmark of notice-and-comment ruling is the requirement that an agency must respond to significant comments in the preamble to the

[9]5 U.S.C. § 553.
[10]Transcript of Oral Argument 25 (June 4, 1990).
[11]*Id.*
[12]*Id.* at 26.
[13]*Id.*

final rule indicating its reasons for rejecting the recommendations set forth in those comments. A rule can be invalidated if the agency's published rationale is not adequate.

The University argued that OSI's procedures violated the APA for two independent reasons. First, the procedures were never published in any form in the *Federal Register*. Second, they were issued without the benefit of notice-and-comment rulemaking. In response, the government argued that OSI's procedures were not actually rules because they only laid out internal procedures for OSI and, therefore, did not affect the substantive rights of citizens. The court rejected that argument noting, among other things, that the procedures set out sanctions and therefore had an effect on persons not in the government. Accordingly, it invalidated the procedures on APA grounds.

With respect to the constitutional claims raised by both Abbs and the University, the court ruled that the interests implicated by the government's action were not of the type that would trigger the due process requirements of the Fifth Amendment. Before an agency is required to afford traditional due process protections (e.g., trial-like hearing), the agency action must threaten either liberty or property interests. The court concluded that Abbs had no property interest at stake because he was not the grantee. Correspondingly, the court ruled that the University, although it was the grantee, had no property interest that was threatened by the investigation. In particular, the court observed that if the government had sought to terminate Abbs' extant grant, then, under the Department's regulations, the University would be entitled to an administrative hearing. However, because OSI lacked the authority to terminate the grant, any concern over the vitality of the grant was speculative.

Abbs also claimed that he had a constitutionally protected liberty interest in continued funding, in continued good standing as a researcher, and in maintaining his personal and scientific reputation. The court held that none of these interests rises to a level to warrant constitutional protection. The court also rejected the University's liberty interest claim as being too speculative.

Both sides have filed notices of appeal with the United States Court of Appeals for the Seventh Circuit and the matter is currently pending before that court. In the meantime, the Public Health Service, in an apparent attempt to blunt the impact of the *Abbs* decision, published a Notice in the June 13, 1991, issue of the *Federal Register* seeking comment on its misconduct procedures. (See "Policies and Procedures for Dealing with Possible Scientific Misconduct in Extramural Research," 56 Fed. Reg. 27,384 (June 13, 1991)). Unfortunately, that Notice falls woefully short of satisfying the requirements of the APA. The APA requires that before a rule is issued the agency must publish a Notice of Proposed Rulemaking (NPRM). An NPRM must be approved by the Office of Management and Budget in the White House and signed by the Secretary of the Department. The PHS Notice was not an NPRM, but rather a mere "Notice." It was not approved by OMB and not signed by the Secretary. In short, the PHS has once again demonstrated an apparent inability to adhere to fundamental principles of administrative law.

Scene 2: Whistle-blowing for Profit

The second case, *United States ex rel. Condie v. the Board of Regents of the University of California, the University of Utah and Ninnemann*, (Civ. Action C-89-3550 (RHS) (N. D. Cal.)) although not directly involving OSI, is potentially far more significant to the research community and the federal government than *Abbs*. The misconduct rules, in theory, were designed to strike a delicate balance between oversight by universities of the research conducted on their campuses and federal stewardship of grant funds. Thus, the self-policing mechanism mandated by section 493 is grounded on the assumption that scientific disputes are best resolved by those with requisite training to evaluate the research in question. *Ex rel. Condie* threatens this delicate balance and seeks, with the blessing of the Department of Justice, to permit these cases to be resolved by lay jurors.

Ex rel. Condie arose under the so-called *qui tam* provisions of the False Claims Amendments Act of 1986.[14] Those provisions authorize any individual, acting as a private attorney general, to institute suit in a federal district court to recover on behalf of the United States monies fraudulently paid to contractors and grantees. Once a suit is filed, the Department of Justice is given the opportunity to intervene on behalf of the plaintiff (technically referred to as the "relator") and to take over the litigation. If the Department of Justice declines to

[14]31 U.S.C. §§ 3729 *et seq.*

intervene, the relator may continue to prosecute the case on behalf of the government. In either event, though, should the relator or government prevail, the relator is entitled to receive a substantial reward (up to 30% of treble the damages suffered by the government as a result of the defendant's fraudulent conduct, if the government declines to intervene).

The False Claims Amendments originally were designed to assit the federal government in weeding out fraud and abuse in defense- related contracts. The law is sufficiently broad, however, to encompass improper conduct by grantees.

In *Ex rel. Condie*, the relator asserted that Ninnemann, a researcher originally employed by the University of Utah and then by the University of California at San Diego, conducted fraudulent research and used that research to obtain NIH grant support. Here Condie is claiming not only that the research was fraudulent, but also that the University of California should have known that it was fraudulent. As a result, the argument goes, the University, as the grantee, submitted a "false claim" and is therefore liable under the Act for treble damages. In August 1990, the Department of Justice, after reviewing the record and consulting with OSI, announced that it would intervene on behalf of Condie. OSI, which had been investigating Ninnemann for some time, temporarily stayed its investigation pending the outcome of the civil suit.

Ex rel. Condie raises a number of intriguing legal issues. For example, is a university now obligated to verify the authenticity of studies that are cited in a grant application? Is a university now liable for monetary damages if it incorrectly determines after conducting an internal investigation that a researcher did not engage in misconduct? These are just a few of the issues likely to surface in *Ex rel. Condie*.

Qui tam actions are not the best nor the most efficient method for resolving cases of misconduct. However, it is now likely that whistleblowers who are dissatisifed with the pace or outcome of an OSI or university investigation will seriously consider *qui tam* actions. In short, the False Claims Amendments place a new premium on efficiency and fairness. Unfortunately, OSI's extant procedures and those of some universities may not be up to the task.

TOWARD A DENOUEMENT

The dramatic tension in the law's response to allegations of fraud in science derives from two profound and countervailing risks.

One is the risk that untrue findings will be grafted onto the corpus of scientific knowledge. Spurious information slows the pursuit of basic knowledge in a singularly pernicious way, and misdirects those who would apply scientific knowledge for human betterment. Wasted time and pilfered national wealth are not the most harmful of the potential consequences. The debasement of the temple of truth is more reprehensible because such desecration can be committed only by its own priests, whose lives ostensibly have been dedicated to the search for truth.

So destructive to the scientific enterprise are these transgressions that the scientist who commits them is never again trusted to do research. Thus, counterpoised against the social harm that may be done by fraud is the risk of permanent personal harm to individual scientists wrongly accused of misconduct. An erroneous finding of misconduct condemns to death an innocent person's career. Moreover, that person's future (and often past) contributions to knowlege are lost irretrievably.

Whereas correct verdicts sentence a scientific sinner to a fitting punishment and strengthen the growing body of knowledge, erroneous acquittals expose the scientific enterprise to further peril and erroneous convictions wrongly destroy careers.

Resolving such terrible dilemmas justly and with minimum error is precisely the task the legal process has been engaged in for centuries. Although the present discussion has been about applications of legal process to problems of science, the methods of science have also been applied to testing alternative legal processes.

Such research has distinguished between conflicts in which the primary issue is a cognitive (or factual) dispute and those in which the principal conflict is one of distributive or attributional justice. Most disputes faced by the law, including those that have been the subject of this chapter, present mixed cases, with justice issues predominating and factual issues cast in a supporting role (Thibaut & Walker, 1978).

Empirical studies of alternative processes for resolving justice disputes consistently find that the process employed makes a considerable difference to the perception of parties and others that the procedure was fair and to their satisfaction with and acceptance of the outcome (Lind & Tyler, 1988; Thibaut & Walker, 1975). When a dispute is brought to a third party for resolution, the more the process used permits the disputants to control the presentation of their respective cases to the fact finder, the better the process and its outcome are received both by winners and losers. Among systems involving third-party resolution, such control is provided more by traditional adversary proceedings than by inquisitorial procedures (wherein the fact finder rather than the parties controls the search for evidence). Where the inquiry follows ad hoc and unpredictable steps, rather than a formal plan, dissatisfaction almost certainly would be still worse. The FDA's procedures compared with those of the NIH clearly reflect what one would expect based on the results of this research. Moreover, although research on procedural justice has, almost by definition, been less interested in questions of accuracy and consistency in fact-finding, other research suggests that traditional legal processes also perform far more impressively on that score than is widely assumed (Saks, 1988).

The discovery of effective legal responses to allegations of scientific misconduct might themselves benefit from the findings of research and theory on dispute resolution.[15] These seem to suggest, along with our tale of two agencies, that more would be less: more legal formalities at the agency stage might produce fewer legal entanglements in courts. Or the legal responses of federal agencies might at least be organized and conducted so as to invite the scrutiny of empirical evaluation. Doing so is likely to hasten the achievement of workable and effective responses.

REFERENCES

Abbs and The Board of Regents of the University of Wisconsin v. Sullivan et al., 756 F. Supp. 1172 (W.D. Wis. 1990).

[15]As this chapter makes clear, the struggle for a suitable process in ongoing. The most recently published hearings are those of the House Committee on Energy and Commerce, Subcommittee on Oversight and Investigations (1990).

Broad, W., & Wade, N. (1982). *Betrayers of the truth*. New York: Simon and Schuster.

House Committee on Energy and Commerce, Subcommittee on Oversight and Investigations. (1988). *Fraud in NIH grant programs: Hearing before the Subcommittee on Oversight and Investigations of the Committee on Energy and Commerce, House of Representatives*, 100th Cong., 2nd sess., April 12, 1988. Washington, DC: United States Congress.

House Committee on Energy and Commerce, Subcommittee on Oversight and Investigations. (1989). *Scientific fraud: Hearings before the Subcommittee on Oversight and Investigations of the Committee on Energy and Commerce, House of Representatives*, 101st Cong., 1st sess., May 4 and 9, 1989. Washington, DC: United States Congress.

House Committee on Energy and Commerce, Subcommittee on Oversight and Investigations. (1990). *Maintaining the integrity of scientific research: Summary of a hearing before the Subcommittee on Investigations and Oversight transmitted to the Committee on Science, Space, and Technology, U.S. House of Representatives*, 101st Cong., 2nd sess. Washington, DC: United States Congress.

House Committee on Government Operations, Human Resources and Intergovernmental Relations Subcommittee. (1988). *Scientific fraud and misconduct and the federal response: Hearing before a Subcommittee on the Committee on Government Operations, House of Representatives*, 100th Cong., 2nd sess., April 11, 1988 and September 29, 1988. Washington, DC: United States Congress.

Kelsey, F. O. (1978). Biomedical monitoring. *Journal of Clinical Pharmacology, 18*, 3–9.

Lind, E. A., & Tyler, T. (1988). *The Social Psychology of Procedural Justice*. New York: Plenum.

National Institutes of Health. (1986). Guide for Grants and Contracts. Bethesda, MD: NIH.

Office of Scientific Integrity. (1990, June 4). Statement of Alan Price, *Transcript of a Special Scientific Panel in re: University of Wisconsin* (June 4, 199), p. 3.

O'Reilly, J. T. (1990). More gold and more fleece: Improving the legal sanctions against medical research fraud. *Administrative Law Review, 42*, 393–422.

Olswang, S. G., & Lee, B. A. (1984). Scientific misconduct: Institutional procedures and due process considerations. *The Journal of College and University Law, 11*, 51–63.

Saks, M. J. (1988). Enhancing and restraining accuracy in adjudication. *Law and Contemporary Problems, 51*, 243–279.

Shapiro, M. F., & Charrow, R. P. (1985). Scientific misconduct in investigational drug trials. *New England Journal of Medicine*, *312*, 731–736.

Shapiro, M. F., & Charrow, R. P. (1989). The role of data audits in detecting scientific misconduct. *Journal of the American Medical Association*, *261*, 2505–2511.

Thibaut, J., & Walker, L. (1975). *Procedural justice: A psychological analysis*. Hillsdale, NJ: Erlbaum.

Thibaut, J., & Walker, L. (1978). A theory of procedure. *Southern California Law Review*, *66*, 541–566.

Van de Kamp, J., & Cummings, M. (1987). *Misconduct and fraud in the life sciences: January 1977 through September 1987*. Bethesda, MD: National Institutes of Health.

Woolf, P. K. (1988). Deception in scientific research. *Jurimetrics Journal*, *29*, 67–95.

The Human Investigator Factor

Cardiology: The John Darsee Experience

EUGENE BRAUNWALD, MD

INTRODUCTION

In August 1989, Drs. David Miller and Michael Hersen wrote me to ask if I would contribute a chapter to this book on the research misconduct of Dr. John Darsee (JD) during his career at Notre Dame (1966–1970), Emory University (1974–1979), and Harvard Medical School (1979–1981), and the discovery and response to JD's misconduct while he was at Harvard in 1981. The editors told me that they hoped I would be willing to share lessons I had drawn from my exposure to this case, now that a decade had passed since the events in question. The JD case is a tragic one, and I have not chosen

The author gratefully acknowledges the cooperation of Dr. Robert L. Kloner, and Messrs. Bancroft N. Littlefield and Robert S. Sanoff in the preparation of this manuscript.

previously to compile the several reports that were written about it at the time into one comprehensive report. But after 10 years, progress had been made on how institutions handle scientific misconduct, more people are aware of how complex these cases can be, I have had some distance on the events, and it seemed appropriate that I agree to the editors' request. Because of highly publicized cases, such as JD's, institutions have become much more sensitive to the possibility of research misconduct. Some institutions, including Harvard Medical School, have adopted written guidelines and rules for addressing allegations of scientific fraud.

Despite the publicity, most scientists still do not appreciate just how difficult investigation of scientific misconduct can be. However, it is now clear to me that I was unprepared to manage what became essentially a full-scale legal, quasi-prosecutorial investigation, and that as a result the initial stages of the matter could have been handled better. I have learned that outside uninvolved parties must be brought in immediately upon the discovey of suspicion of misconduct, and that once any *hard* evidence of misconduct is discovered the burden switches to the accused scientist to prove that his other research is accurate. I have also learned that advisers experienced in conducting such investigations, interviewing witnesses, and walking what may be a fine line between obligation to science and the individual's right to due process should be consulted at the earliest opportunity.

The following report summarizes the facts involved in the JD case and offers several general reflections concerning scientific misconduct. The summary is basically a compilation of materials submitted to the National Heart, Lung and Blood Institute (NHLBI) in 1981 and 1982 and of the reports by the Ad Hoc Advisory Committee to the Dean of the Harvard Medical School (HMS) (1982), the Special Panel of the National Heart, Lung and Blood Institute (1982), and two reports of committees at Emory University (1983a, 1983b).

EVENTS PRECEDING MAY 1981

JD was born in Huntington, West Virginia, in 1948. He attended the University of Notre Dame and his curriculum vitae states that he was on the Dean's list between 1967 and 1970. During his junior year at Notre Dame JD published, as sole author, two papers in *The Notre*

Dame Science Quarterly. He graduated with a B.S. in 1970. He then attended Indiana University School of Medicine from which he received the M.D. in 1974. JD was strongly recommended by Indiana University for graduate medical training, which he took at Emory University. From 1974 to 1977 he served a medical internship and residency and then was a Clinical Fellow in Cardiology. His performance in these roles was considered to be exemplary by his supervising faculty, and he was selected to be Chief Resident in Medicine at Grady Memorial Hospital and Instructor in Medicine at Emory from 1978 to 1979. In 1978 he won the Lloyd Hyde Research Competition and in 1979 three additional awards, including first place in a Basic Science Research Forum sponsored by the American College of Chest Physicians. During his training as a resident and chief Resident in Medicine and Fellow in Cardiology at Emory, JD was extremely prolific and authored several dozen articles and chapters in textbooks and manuals and several dozen abstracts.

In 1977, JD applied for a Research Fellowship in the Cardiac Research Laboratory of the HMS and the Brigham and Women's Hospital (BWH) to commence in July, 1979. He was accepted on the basis of two personal interviews with me and another member of the faculty; a strong verbal recommendation from the Chairman of the Department of Medicine at Emory; and three strong letters of recommendation that followed, from senior members of the faculty at Emory. These letters, which were written in January and February 1978 (i.e., almost a year and a half before he came to Boston and before his Chief Residency in Medicine), were unusually laudatory. Thus, one Professor wrote:

. . . I am writing in support of Dr. John Darsee's application for a research fellowship in your Cardiology Program (1979–80).

I have followed John's progress in our training programs closely and am serving as a research advisor for several projects that he has underway. He is clearly one of the most intelligent, energetic and hard working individuals in the Medicine Department's Programs. *In ten years of working with medical students, house officers, and cardiology trainees, both in my basic science laboratory (Physiology) and on clinical research projects (Cardiology Service) I have not encountered anyone with more curiosity, enthusiasm or potential for developing into an excellent investigator. He can convert clinical research projects, can collect data rapidly and carefully, and then analyze, synthesize and write with considerable ability and clarity* [my emphasis]. . . .

Another senior faculty member wrote:

. . . His performance as a house officer in Internal Medicine and as a Fellow in Cardiology has been extraordinary. He is very bright, but, of course, so are other medical house officers. Few medical trainees, however, have the amazing self discipline and drive that John possesses. . . . *John is better suited for a career in academic medicine than anyone that I have seen in the cardiology training program at Emory University in the past few years* [my emphasis]. His greatest strength is an unusually fine blend of intelligence, self discipline, ambition and personality. If this letter is interpreted as simply just another non-discriminatory note of praise, I will have done John a disservice. He is truly outstanding. I have not recommended a candidate so highly in years!. . .

A third Professor wrote:

. . . John has been engaged in several research projects, which he has pursued regularly and doggedly, not allowing his clinical responsibilities to interfere with his research efforts nor his research efforts to interfere with his clinical responsibilities. His energy seems boundless, as does his ability. He has the maturity, well beyond his years, to define the boundaries of a problem that will make it amenable to answering, to acquire the techniques necessary to solve the problem, and then to go about so doing in a precise, methodological manner. . . .

In July, 1979 he began his training as a Research Fellow in the Cardiac Research Laboratory, which was under my overall direction and under the day-to-day supervision of Dr. Robert Koner (RK), who at the time was an Assistant Professor of Medicine at HMS and an Established Investigator of the American Heart Association. Prior to assuming these responsibilities, RK had earned both the MD and PhD degrees, and had received training in cardiovascular research in three separate laboratories over 7 years. Although he (RK) had some clinical responsibilities, most of his time was spent in the laboratory working closely and on a daily basis with three or four post-doctoral fellows (including JD) and the technical staff. I too had close contact with JD throughout the 2 years of his Fellowship, meeting with him or

RK regularly and frequently to review data from the laboratory and to plan experiments.

JD's research was on the reduction of infarct size by pharmacologic agents in dogs with experimentally induced coronary occlusion; his salary was supported by an NIH individual postdoctoral research fellowship (NRSA), a peer-reviewed competitive award. JD's work in our laboratory appeared to be exemplary, and we agreed with his former mentors at Emory that he was indeed unusually capable. His research productivity as HMS–BWH was also outstanding. During the first 22 months he was the first author of seven original papers published in quality scientific journals. JD worked prodigiously, 90–100 hours per week; he contributed good ideas about the research in which he was engaged, read avidly, was excellent with his hands, a good experimental surgeon, and a fine physiologist with a flair for applying electronics in the laboratory. He brought to the laboratory expertise in the measurement of instantaneous cardiac dimensions by means of sonocardiometry, a technique which he had learned at Emory. Moreover, JD was pleasant, neat, and personable; he was a positive influence, making constructive suggestions about laboratory organizations and procedures.

JD rapidly became more adept in experimentation and, in accord with the laboratory's policies, assumed responsibility commensurate with his increasing skills. For example, once it was clear to RK and me that JD could accurately make the measurements required in a particular experiment, an increasing proportion of the time we spent with him was devoted to discussing experimental design and results.

In the Spring of 1981, several months before the scheduled completion of his postdoctoral fellowship, JD informed me that he had been invited to return to a very attractive position as a faculty member in the Department of Medicine at Emory. Based on his superb performance in our laboratory, we also offered him a faculty position in the Cardiovascular Division of the Department of Medicine at the Beth Israel Hospital. I had agreed to nominate him for an Assistant Professorship of Medicine at HMS commencing July 1, 1981. Indeed, at the very time that the first evidence of his research misconduct came to light in May 1981, I was still receiving glowing letters of recommendation about JD from the faculty at Emory. These letters, by some of the same respondents who had initially recommended JD for his Fellowship with us, remained unusually complimentary. Indeed, they were written three years after the first set and were based on additional exposure to JD. Thus, one respondent wrote:

> . . . Despite an enormous commitment to teaching and patient care, John continued to collaborate and produce first class scientific publications throughout his remaining 3 years at Emory. He was a stimulus to all around him, and his knowledge and teaching sessions were sought after by all of those around him. He is warm and friendly, and is a true humanitarian. *I have no doubt that John is one of the leading internist-cardiologists of his age group in the country* [my emphasis]. . . .

Another wrote:

> . . . When I wrote to you several years ago in support of Dr. John Darsee's application for a fellowship in cardiovascular research, I said that he was extraordinary. The past two years have only reinforced that view.
>
> *Dr. Darsee is clearly one of the most remarkable young men in American medicine* [my emphasis]. There is little need to dwell on his accomplishments in cardiovascular research. His curriculum vitae offers abundant evidence that he does original work, and that he does it in great abundance.
>
> Dr. Darsee has achieved a national reputation within a few short years, a fact that places him in a rather elite group.
>
> I am equally impressed by Dr. Darsee's performance outside the research laboratory. He has demonstrated excellent clinical skills and teaching ability. It is not extravagant to say that *Dr. Darsee became a legendary figure during his year as Chief Resident in Medicine* [my emphasis] at Grady Memorial Hospital. . . .

THE EVENTS OF MAY 1981

In the early spring of 1981 the other two postdoctoral research fellows in the Cardiac Research Laboratory became suspicious of the veracity of JD's research and wondered whether he was actually producing all of the data he claimed. Because of lack of firm evidence, they did not bring their suspicions to anyone's attention. However, in the middle of May 1981, they, as well as the senior technician, were shocked to observe JD fabricating data. Specifically he was observed to be labeling recordings that he was making on an instrumented dog, "24 hours," "72 hours," "one week," and "two weeks," with only seconds or minutes between obtaining these tracings. On the next day JD presented these tracings to RK as valid data to be included in an abstract. The fellows and technician informed RK, who immediately carried out a careful investigation of the matter, confronted JD with the evidence of data fabrication, and on May 22, 1981, came to me with the disturbing evidence and conclusion that JD had indeed fabricated data to be included in an abstract that he wished to submit to be presented before the Scientific Sessions of the American Heart Association and to be published. On the next working day, I separately interviewed all of the aforementioned and confirmed RK's conclusion. I then met with JD and told him of the accusations. He immediately admitted his guilt, gave no satisfactory explanation for the flagrant misconduct, apologized profusely, and insisted that he had never engaged in any other irregularity of research practice. I pointed out the seriousness of the situation, immediately withdrew the offer of a faculty appointment at HMS, and informed him that it would be necessary to conduct a detailed investigation of all of his other research activities in the laboratory. JD stated that he welcomed the review and agreed to cooperate fully. I informed the Dean for Academic Affairs of HMS of this matter by telephone and the Dean of HMS, as well as the President of the BWH, in writing. I told JD that his NIH National Research Service Award and his Research Fellowships at HMS and the BWH would have to be terminated, which they were, effective June 30, 1981. However, I asked JD to stay in the Boston area in an informal capacity for several months, in part to assist us with the verification process.

In our initial investigation, during the course of the next few days and weeks, it was not clear whether this had been a single inexcusable event, an impulsive act performed by a talented person in a fit of anger or working under some pressure, as JD claimed, or whether it was part of a broader pattern of misconduct. RK and I felt, of course, that it was vital to assure ourselves of the validity (or lack thereof) of all other data obtained by JD. In addition to protecting the integrity of the scientific process, our reputations, and that of JD's other co-workers, we felt that it was essential to determine the extent of JD's misdeeds consonant with the due process which we believed JD was entitled to receive. Upon completion of the investigation we hoped that he could be dealt with justly and counseled properly and that prospective employers and granting agencies could be accurately informed. Accordingly, RK and I, singly and together, spent many hours reviewing individual experiments carried out by JD since his arrival in the laboratory in July 1979 and initially found nothing that was suspicious.

The abstract at issue, which started the investigation and which, of course, was never submitted, actually was not based on a study planned or formally sponsored by the laboratory; rather, it was based on observations JD claimed to have made and then confirmed by a series of further experiments designed to test a hypothesis resulting from them. The fabrication apparently occurred after RK requested JD to produce the raw data and tracings from these experiments, in accord with the well-established laboratory practice of reviewing the original data before submission. It was soon after this request that JD was observed to label tracings of several hours' duration as having been recorded over several weeks. JD claimed to have performed the experiments appropriately weeks earlier, but because he had been assigned a new desk and storage cabinets he could not locate the original records. Given these facts, it looked initially as if the fabrication might indeed have occurred in response to a unique set of circumstances—JD's rush to submit his abstract by the mid-May deadline and his need to have sufficient raw data to pass RK's scrutiny.

THE MODELS STUDY

Prior to May 1981, JD and RK had been involved in a blinded, multicenter, randomized study organized by the NHLBI, termed the Models Study. The experiments were not quite completed at the end of May 1981. JD had been responsible for the dog surgery, the injection of radioisotopes, and the analysis of myocardial samples for radioactivity for the measurement of regional myocardial blood flow; RK had been responsible for the histology, histochemistry, and estimation of infarct size. The study had been carried out for many months and involved three other laboratories in other Universities. Most of the experiments were carried out prior to the end of May 1981 (i.e., prior to the initial discovery of JD's misdeed). All four laboratories participating in the Models Study submitted their interim results to the NHLBI in April 1981, and neither we nor anyone else was notified that something might be amiss. We permitted JD to complete his portion of the Models experiments after May 22 but under closer supervision; the last experiment which he performed was on July 25, 1981. An important purpose of allowing JD to complete the experiments was to determine whether RK and I could have confidence in the work he had carried out prior to May 1981, especially on the Model's study. It was felt that careful observation of JD during these weeks and comparison of the results obtained by him prior to and after May might aid in the resolution of these issues. This hunch proved to be correct.

As results of individual experiments in the Models study were reviewed by RK and me, nothing out of the ordinary was found at first. However, when, during the last week of October 1981, we saw the graphs of the results of all of the experiments—not only those from our laboratory but those of the other investigators as well—we noted that the regional myocardial blood flow data provided by JD showed an unexpected, perhaps unbelievably, low degree of variability. Some of the other investigators in the study also became concerned with the data at this time, as did NHLBI staff. On October 30, at a meeting of the investigators involved in the Models Study and NHLBI staff, RK alerted the attendees and expressed our concern with the validity of these results. The graphs provided at this meeting by the NHLBI were further analyzed, and a comparison of the results of experiments performed by JD prior to and after May 22, 1981 (the date that JD's fabrication of data was established) was performed and indicated a marked difference.

When confronted with the graphs and the unlikely low variability in blood flow in the first 35 (pre-May 22) experiments, JD steadfastly denied any wrongdoing. It had been his practice to analyze for radioactivity the samples of myocardium for the measurement of regional blood flow in a scintillation counter in a building other than that in which the Cardiac Research Laboratory was located, and from these counts he claimed to have calculated the values of regional myocardial blood flow in his laboratory notebooks. When we asked him to provide the original printouts from the scintillation counter he said that he had discarded them because of lack of filing space. Because RK and I could not stand behind the measurements of myocardial blood flow, we formally withdrew our results from the multicenter study and informed NHLBI staff and officials as well as the coinvestigators of our concerns with the regional flow data in a letter dated November 3, 1981. The discrepancies between pre-May 22 and post-May 22 results in JD's blood flow and heart weight data led us to conclude that JD's misconduct must have extended beyond the single admitted fabrication.

EXPERIMENTS IN THE RADIOLOGY DEPARTMENT

Shortly after his arrival in Boston in July 1979, JD, with my knowledge, commenced training and a collaborative relation with a faculty member in the Department of Radiology. JD continued experiments in this investigator's laboratory without informing him that he no longer held HMS or BWH appointments. Early in November 1981 I was surprised to learn that this collaboration had continued and that they had submitted two manuscripts, one of which, in fact had already been accepted for publication. I immediately reviewed these papers, and in one of them found correlations that, on the basis of my experience with the methods employed, were so good that they strained credulity. I sought advice on this matter from an expert in another institution and he agreed with my skepticism. I informed my colleague in the Department of Radiology about my suspicions and he accepted my recommendation that he withdraw the two papers. He informed me that subsequent analysis indicated that the results of one of these two studies, in which JD had no control of the data, were valid, whereas serious questions remained unanswered about the validity of the second, which had also troubled me. Subsequently, the Ad Hoc Advisory Committee to the Dean of the Harvard Medical School on Dishonesty in Scientific Research and the NHLBI Panel confirmed that JD had indeed engaged in fabrication of research data in the Radiology Department.

INQUIRIES FROM PROSPECTIVE EMPLOYERS

In the summer and fall of 1981 we had received two telephone inquiries about JD, who by this time had applied for academic positions in other institutions. We informed the two prospective employers, Professors of Medicine and Directors of Cardiology at other institutions, that JD had committed and admitted research misconduct and that we had withdrawn the offer of a position on our faculty for that specific reason. In addition, in November 1981 I informed the Chairman of Medicine and the Chief of Cardiology of Emory University, JD's former mentors, of the entire matter. I recommended that they institute the kind of verification procedures that we were employing on JD's research from Emory which was published, or which was then in press.

DISCOVERY OF ADDITIONAL MISCONDUCT IN BOSTON

During the winter of 1981 and the spring of 1982 RK and I continued to investigate JD's research practices. The Cardiac Research Laboratory maintained a list of disposal of dogs that had been rendered radioactive by the injection of isotopes in order to measure regional myocardial blood flow. We discovered discrepancies between the radioactive dog disposal list maintained by the laboratory technicians, and JD's laboratory notebooks, throwing into question whether dogs that JD claimed to have given radioisotopes actually received them. Following this new lead, we made the startling discovery that blocks of tissue obtained from hearts now approximately a year old, into which JD had claimed he had injected radioactive microspheres, did not in fact contain any residual radioactivity; the latter should have been easily detected even after one year with the sensitive analytic methods that were employed. On the other hand, tissue from dogs in the Models Study operated on by JD after May 22, 1981 (after his initial misconduct had been discovered), contained substantial residual radioactivity. These observations were followed up by microscopic analysis of the tissue, which confirmed the presence of microspheres in the post-May 22 hearts, but none in the pre-May 22 hearts. We shared these findings with HMS and NIH and obtained independent verification of their accuracy. This evidence, for which we had been searching for months, was the strongest proof of misconduct since JD had made his original admission on the single abstract in May 1981. From May 1981 JD clung steadfastly to his denial of any misdeed other than the single event that he had admitted in May 1981.

It is interesting that this *definitive* evidence of serious wrongdoing by JD came from a straightforward and simple analysis of radioactivity in tissue samples, yet it took us so long to focus on it. None of the many experts who had been deeply involved in looking at this matter, including authorities in radioisotopes, pathology, and cardiovascular physiology, thought of carrying out these determinations; yet it was clear to all who asked that the tissue in question was still available.

THE HARVARD INVESTIGATION

In November 1981 the Dean of HMS and I independently concluded that because of the increasing complexity of this matter it would be desirable for an ad hoc committee, drawn from responsible senior members of the academic community, both from Harvard University and outside, to develop a statement of the facts of the case and make recommendations for handling this (and other similar) case(s). Such a committee (Ad Hoc Advisory Committee to the Dean of HMS on Dishonesty in Scientific Research) was appointed in November 1981 and delivered its initial report on January 25, 1982.

A Subcommittee of the ad hoc committee conducted a site visit of the Cardiovascular Research Laboratory in December 1981 and "reviewed the systems for data collection and preservation used by Dr. Darsee and other members of the laboratory." The Committee stated:

[T]he Subcommittee visiting the laboratory and the Committee as a whole were convinced that the laboratory directed by Dr. Kloner was well administered with appropriate regard to data collection and review. The visiting Subcommittee noted that data books dating back to 1977 revealed an "impressive set of well maintained, annotated and stored raw data that was in good enough condition to allow reanalysis even at this time and seemed complete with protocol, mathematical analysis and finished conclusions." The Subcommittee concluded that: "the present problem does not appear to be at all referable to the existing Cardiac Research Laboratory standards, policies or procedures, nor to overt pressure provided by its director of Dr. Braunwald. Dr. Robert Kloner and the Cardiac Research Laboratory have maintained an extremely effective system for data collection, analysis and storage."

The Ad Hoc Committee stated:

When considered in two phases, the responses of the institution seem reasonable in relation to the information available at the respective times. The first phase response was prompt, but limited, and seemed appropriate for what then appeared to be a single episode of aberrant behavior. The realization that there might be more than one episode of dishonesty appropriately precipitated the larger and more comprehensive second phase response in November and December.

The committee questioned the reason for the delay between the initial event and response in May and June and the fullscale investigation in November. In retrospect, it is clear that Drs. Braunwald and Kloner felt in May and June that they were probably dealing with a single bizarre act by a young man who had performed exceptionally well previously. In the light of this consideration, the plan selected in June seems to be reasonable in that it provided an opportunity to assess the extent of the damage and also to provide for a period of observation under supervision. . .

The Committee suggested two ways in which the institution's response to the problem could have been improved:

. . . First, a small committee of senior professors from within the University, but outside the involved department, should have been consulted immediately after the discovery in May. (Perhaps there should be a standing committee to deal with such matters.) In any case, such a committee, be it standing or ad hoc, could have shared the burden with the Dean, the Chairman of the Department, and the Laboratory Director and offered objective advice concerning the management of the problem. The second suggestion has to do with internal communication. In May a systematic search should have been conducted to identify all persons within the institution with whom Dr. Darsee had collaborated, and these persons should have been informed confidentially of the allegations brought against him. . .

The Committee also raised a number of broader questions about the conduct of biomedical science and made a number of important suggestions such as (1) the desirability for a greater emphasis on the quality rather than the quantity of publications in academic promotions; (2) the desirability that national societies limit the number of abstracts submitted by a single author; (3) and the responsibilities of institutions discovering dishonesty in research to other institutions, to the scientific and medical communities, and to the public. The Committee also suggested a number of specific steps regarding how the institution should deal with any future such occurrences.

THE NHLBI PANEL

In December 1981 the NHLBI appointed a panel of four "senior investigators with extensive experience in cardiovascular research" from outside Harvard to "review [the] alleged misconduct. . . the circumstances and the corrective actions taken, or yet to be taken. . . ." The panel was aided by a staff of 10 staff members from NIH, including science administrators, statisticians, and attorneys. The panel carried out site visits, examined data and records, interviewed all relevant parties including JD, and obtained multiple computer-generated analyses of relevant data. The panel's report was released in February 1983 and stated:

> . . . apart from the professional misconduct of Dr. John Darsee, the integrity and scientific capabilities of the professional and technical staff of the Cardiovascular Laboratory at the Brigham and Women's Hospital are of a high order. . . none of the Panel's findings suggest the involvement of any individual other than Dr. Darsee in the data fabrication at the Brigham and Women's laboratory. . . .

> . . . Hospital officials complied with their legal obligations, and there were no official NIH guidelines indicating that they should have informed NIH [of their reasons for terminating the fellowship of Dr. Darsee].

Similarly, the Report acknowledges that

> . . . NIH has not issued guidelines concerning the responsibility of grantees, sponsors, or contractors to report actual or alleged misconduct. . .

> The [Cardiac Research] Laboratory has had an outstanding record of productivity since its establishment by Dr. Braunwald in 1973. It has provided research training and experience for many young investigators. . . . In many respects supervision in the Cardiac Research Labo-

ratory. . . has been adequate and comparable to that provided in similar laboratories at other institutions.

In addition, the Report noted that "as a consequence of Dr. Darsee's misconduct, this laboratory has undergone an unusually rigorous scrutiny." It stated:

> General supervisory practices [in the Cardiac Research Laboratory] have been based, appropriately, on an assumption of honesty and trust between supervisors and trainees. With the exception of Dr. Darsee, recent trainees have retained original records in customary and acceptable fashion. They have been allowed appropriately increasing independence as their laboratory experience has progressed. Because most incoming trainees have had superior records of previous accomplishment, they have perhaps been capable of progressing more rapidly than trainees in many other laboratories.

> Drs. Braunwald and Kloner deserve full credit for initiating the measurement of residual radioactivity in cardiac tissues. This technique led to the important discovery that there was an absence of residual radioactivity in many of the hearts in which Dr. Darsee purported to have measured myocardial blood flow by injecting radioactive microsphers.

However, the panel was not without criticism of the laboratory and of some of our actions. Among its criticisms was that our initial investigation of JD's work had been "insufficiently rigorous." that "a hurried pace and emphasis on productivity" existed in the laboratory, and that "the supervisory practices in the laboratory, while in no way responsible for Dr. Darsee's misconduct, may have contributed inadvertently to the ease with which he was able to produce fabricated data and to the subsequent difficulty in documenting the extent of the problem." The panel also was critical of the decision in May 1981 not to notify the NHLBI when JD's first instance of misconduct came to light and to let JD continue to perform experiments in the Models Study. The panel also indicated that "randomization procedures and some experimental methods [are described] in a manner that does not represent the actual procedures and methods in a completely accurate way."

In the course of the panel's investigation statistical analyses were performed by NHLBI staff that called into question much of the tabular data provided by JD in published papers. In several papers a striking lack of variability was observed in measurements of regional myocardial blood flow among groups of dogs relative to the within-group variability. The reports stated:

> When possible independence of the standard error of the mean and sample size was examined, two papers were found to contain variables for which the standard error of the mean was virtually unchanged for groups with substantially different sample sizes. In regard to the measurement of regional myocardial blood flow, fractional differences between sequential measurements in nonischemic segments in one paper were less than the measurement error of the microsphere technique reported in the literature.

As a consequence of this compelling, albeit indirect evidence, as well as the more direct proof that JD did not inject radioactive substances into dogs for the measurement of regional myocardial blood flow, the papers coauthored by JD in the Cardiac Research Laboratory to which he contributed data were retracted.

Upon receipt of the Panel's report JD was debarred from receiving grant and contract funding from NIH and he was excluded from service on any NIH peer review or program committee, each for a period of 10 years. The funds that had been received for the study were returned to the NIH; the laboratory was revisited one year later and no problems were found.

COMMENT

The Rigor of the Investigation

The NHLBI Panel consisted of a group of distinguished scientists who had substantial resources and a dedicated and competent staff. They had access to all of JD's research materials, tissue specimens, notebooks, and laboratory records, and had full opportunity to interview all relevant parties, including JD. Nevertheless, over the 5 months of its work the Panel and its staff never suggested measuring residual radioactivity in the remaining heart tissue. Therefore, they did not uncover the startling fact and most powerful direct evidence of misconduct that, although he reported that he had done so, JD did *not* in fact inject radioisotopes for the measurement of blood flow in the 35

Model's Study dogs he operated on before May 22, 1981, and in a number of dogs from his published work.

This demonstrates the inherent difficulty of investigating fraudulent scientific data and uncovering conclusive as opposed to circumstantial evidence of misconduct. This difficulty is compounded when the perpetrator refuses to admit misconduct and insists that his research is accurate.

JD's Supervision

Because JD came to HMS and BWH with such high recommendations and was completing his seventh year of postdoctoral training at the time his misconduct was first discovered, it did not appear to RK and me to be necessary (or indeed desirable) to scrutinize his every activity or to recheck all of his primary data. JD was observed by RK and others to be carrying out experiments in the laboratory, analyzing records, and calculating results. He was a prodigious worker who stayed in the laboratory until late at night several times a week and on weekends. He showed and discussed the results of individual experiments with RK almost on a daily basis. Then, at a series of research meetings with RK and me, JD presented the tracings and graphs of results of several experiments. These were reviewed, and plans for further experimentation were developed by RK, JD, and myself. Subsequently, JD was observed to be carrying out experiments by RK, and he returned to RK and me with what appeared to be accurate results.

Why Was JD's Single Act of Misconduct Not Reported to the NHLBI in May 1981?

Of course, had I known in May what I knew in November 1981 of the extent of JD's misconduct, I would have reported it immediately to the NIH and insisted on an external investigation (as I did in November). However, at the time (May 1981) one of my concerns was that JD be treated fairly, and in the absence at that time of relevant guidelines (from NIH, the University, or the Hospital) this led to the decision in May to take no action to publicize the facts surrounding this dismissal from HMS and BWH, although we did cause his NIH fellowships to be terminated at that time. What we knew in May 1981 was that an apparently brilliant researcher had committed and acknowledged a single incident of serious misconduct. Our initial investigation uncovered no evidence of further misconduct.

I determined that there were essentially three kinds of responses available. At one end of the spectrum, JD could have been issued a severe reprimand, placed under observation, and continued at the University, the Hospital, and the Laboratory on probation. At the other end of the spectrum, we could essentially have terminated his academic career. He could have been dismissed from the University and from the Hospital and his single, admitted incident of misconduct could have been made public by, among other such steps, reporting the conduct to the NIH. Channels through which the matter could have been reported to the NIH under an assurance of confidentiality, as are available now, did *not* exist at the time. The middle ground, which I selected, consisted of notifying appropriate University and Hospital authorities immediately, as well as potential employers who made inquiry, withdrawing immediately the offer of a faculty appointment, terminating JD's fellowships at HMS, BWH, and NIH, and beginning an audit of his work, but allowing him to complete experiments in the laboratory for a brief period under closer supervision. This middle course seemed the most reasonable because it appeared at the time that only a single acknowledged act of fraudulently recreating original tracings was involved. When it became evident in October that the scope of JD's misconduct was broader than initially known, I immediately took a series of much more severe steps.

In hindsight, the decision to permit JD to remain in the laboratory and perform experiments in the Models Study under closer supervision appeared to some to have been a mistake. This decision, however, enabled RK and me to compare the results of his experiments pre-May 22, 1981 and post-May 22, and to provide the basis for many subsequent conclusions as to the scope of JD's misconduct.

The Harvard Ad Hoc Committee Report, while recognizing, as do I, that as it turned out there were heavy costs to the decision, made this same point:

As the Committee looks back at the events of the summer and fall of 1981, it appears clear that it was helpful to allow Dr. Darsee to continue working in the laboratory because the comparison of the pre-May 22 and post-May 22 data in the "Models Study" proved to be of great value in the final analysis. On the other hand , this course of action was not without cost. Dr. Darsee's presence in the laboratory environment after the events of May proved to be damaging to the morale and productivity of the laboratory.

THE EMORY INVESTIGATION

In November 1981, as mentioned earlier, I advised the Chairman of Medicine of Emory University of our discoveries of JD's misconduct and urged him to review JD's work there. I did not hear back and in December 1981 I examined several of JD's published papers from Emory University. On the basis of this review, I developed serious questions about the validity of some of the data in these papers from Emory and I reported these questions to JD's former superiors at Emory, as well as to the NHLBI Panel and staff. In February 1982 the Dean of Emory University School of Medicine appointed an Internal Committee to review JD's work at that institution, which had resulted in the publication of 10 research papers and 45 abstracts. This Committee rendered its report in March 1983, and in April 1983 an External (to Emory) Review Committee confirmed and endorsed the report.

The Emory Committee found that although JD enjoyed an excellent reputation at Emory, one faculty member in the Department of Pathology *had, in fact, become suspicious of the veracity of JD's contribution to one study and had informed his superior of the problem.* The Committee found "overwhelming direct and circumstantial evidence of flagrant and extensive fraud" in JD's research at Emory University and of fabrication of data published in the name of the University after he was at Harvard. The Committee found serious problems in eight of these papers, which were ultimately retracted upon the conclusion of its investigation. These problems included the inability to confirm from hospital records the diagnosis in some patients described. Some papers describing human studies had apparently not been submitted to the human investigations committee for approval, and it was questionable if they had ever been performed. Review of some papers revealed totally implausible results, such as those based on having obtained myocardial tissue at autopsy within 4 hours of death in a large number of patients. One published paper was described as coming from Emory and Harvard; review at both institutions indicated that it could not have been carried out at either, and the Committee concluded that the experiments described in the paper must have been fictitious. In several instances, JD placed coauthors on publications without their permission, indeed without their knowledge. In some instances, the coauthors, who were faculty members, did not even know about the project and first became aware of the research at the time of publication of the abstracts. One paper acknowledged the cooperation of physicians and scientists who were apparently nonexistent, and in one published abstract an apparently nonexistent coauthor was listed.

The Committee wrote:

> A pattern of deception, manipulation, of data and of people and outright fabrication of research data now appears to be a truer characterization of this person (JD). . . . One of the papers. . . is the most flagrant example of the fabrication and dissembling that pervades most of the papers and abstracts. A structure was built that would appear to be convincing evidence of the conclusion. . . . Many abstracts were submitted for presentation at national meetings without the knowledge of the "collaborators."

Regarding the abstracts that JD had coauthored, the Committee's Chairman concluded ". . . of the 45 abstracts that are now known only two can be considered to be valid. Many of the abstracts appear to be completely fictitious. . . ."

THE PAPERS AT NOTRE DAME

Shortly after some of the details of the JD affair were widely publicized, I received a letter from a faculty member at Notre Dame, indicating that the two articles that JD published in the student-run *Notre Dame Science Quarterly* in 1969 were almost certainly fabrications. After learning of JD's widespread research misconduct in the popular press, this faculty member carried out a detailed analysis of these two papers and conceded that it was unlikely, indeed impossible, for JD to have done the work described in these two papers. My own review and that of two experts in the field (endocrinology) of these two papers, indicated that they could not have been carried out as stated.

REFLECTIONS

Although the vast majority of scientists are honest, a small percentage cheat occasionally, usually under great pressure or when they feel that the stakes are very high. By tampering even slightly and only occasionally with the truth, a scientist abuses the special privilege of trust that society bestows on all scientists. Such behavior obviously is not only antisocial; even if it is never discovered it is ultimately counterproductive to the researcher because it bases his career, at least in part, on deception, rather than on the "disinterested, objective search for truth," which is the foundation of all science. On the other hand, like any occasional crime, fraud in science can have short-term benefits to the perpetrator—such as the acceptance of a paper by a prestigious journal, the awarding of a grant, or even an academic promotion.

JD appears not to have been a scientist (in training) engaged in only occasional misconduct. Instead, the evidence indicates that he provided false research data continuously over a period of many years—from his college days at Notre Dame, through his years at Emory, and finally in two separate laboratories at HMS and BWH, until his misconduct was discovered in the Cardiac Research Laboratory and as a consequence was finally exposed. It appears that JD's research misconduct from the very beginning was pervasive, limited only by what he thought the system in which he worked would tolerate. For example, in the Cardiac Research Laboratory at HMS-BWH, the vast bulk of the measurements that he made under close observation (i.e., those that involved surgery on dogs, and physiological measurements such as intracardiac pressure and cardiac dimensions) appear to have been accurate. It was the measurements that he made unobserved, such as those of regional myocardial blood flow, which were fabricated. Even the latter appear to have been obtained honestly and accurately when they were being carefully scrutinized, such as during his first few months in the laboratory, or in the last few Models Study experiments performed in June and July of 1981.

JD was an unusually talented person who had the native intelli-

gence, technical and interpersonal skills, and creativity to be a very
successful physician–scientist, indeed a leader in cardiovascular academic medicine. Sadly, his behavior in the research laboratory was
self-destructive. We must look to the behavioral sciences to help
explain the deeper motivations for the repeated commitment of research fraud, especially when it is as gross and widespread as JD's
was. Because this activity is so detrimental to self, to colleagues, to
institutions, and to science as a whole, I believe that it is a form of
unconscious self-destructive behavior, with aggressive components
directed also toward colleages, supervisors, institutions, and society,
all of whom are profoundly affected. The role played by external
pressures in pervasive as opposed to occasional misconduct is less
clear.

Needless to say, I learned much from this episode. Some of the
lessons are:

1. When a trainee or student is involved in alleged misconduct, the
trainer or teacher, while playing an integral role in the investigation,
should not become one of the decision makers. The responsibilities of
mentoring and advising a trainee and the resultant natural inclination
to be the trainee's advocate can conflict with the equally important
responsibility to unearth the truth, even when the latter can destroy
the trainee's professional life. A group from outside the laboratory,
department, or even institution, is better equipped to deal with the
many competing demands and forces that come into play in such a
matter.

2. I now believe that once a single act of blatant scientific dishonesty is discovered the burden must shift from finding other evidence of
misconduct to proving that the scientist's other data were produced
honestly. While at the time it seemed reasonable to give JD the benefit
of an initial assumption that he might have committed only an isolated
act of misconduct, I believe in retrospect that such an initial assumption was not warranted and delayed the pace and scope of the investigation. In retrospect, JD's outright fabrication of data was so extreme
that I should have assumed that it was part of a more pervasive pattern
of behavior.

3. There should be no surprise that after exhaustive investigations
by a variety of committees, no one else was found guilty of research
misconduct. To my knowledge, no instances of biomedical research

fraud have been uncovered that involved the knowing participation of more than one person (i.e., a conspiracy).

4. The retrospectoscope is a wonderful instrument. Had we known in May 1981 what we knew in October 1981, our actions would have been different. When the JD matter came to light in 1981, there were virtually no guidelines or requirements concerning the reporting of research fraud, proved or suspected. Such guidelines now are available.

The complexity of balancing the interests involved in the JD case and responding to the circumstances as they gradually became known in the absence of guidelines as to how to deal with such a matter is reflected in the testimony of Dr. Donald Frederickson, then Director of the NIH, and the late Dr. Philip Handler, then President of the National Academy of Sciences, before the Congressional Subcommittee on Investigations on Oversight on March 31 and April 1, 1981, less than two months before we discovered JD's misconduct:

DR. FREDERICKSON: to be sure also because human beings are involved; ambitious human beings, seeking honor and prestige and we can easily injure them; we can destroy them for a whole career. We can cast them out of science and *one has to be extraordinarily careful in the exercise of judgment and the kind of justice that is harsh* [my emphasis] and exists in dealing with these matters.

MR. GORE: Did you wish to comment, Dr. Handler?

DR. HANDLER: I just couldn't agree more with what Dr. Frederickson has just said. But I will admit with you, sir, the absence of any sense of what due process should be when some suspicion is aroused. *We have never adopted standardized procedures of any kind to deal with these isolated events. We have no courts, no sets of courts, no understandings among ourselves as to how any one such incident shall be treated* [my emphasis].

We have left them, one at a time, as they have occurred, to the best judgment of the institutions within which such events have transpired when one thought they had. And, in the end, word of such misdeeds which attaches to the name of the individual invariably destroys him in the career on which he had embarked. We think that suffices; more than suffices

Later in the same hearing:

DR. FREDERICKSON: Nothing like that [the discrediting of a scientist involved in data falsification] moves immediately. I don't think you get that speed. It moves very deliberately, because one must be sure. *If the result is the exclusion of that individual from science, that is the ultimate penalty, and one must proceed carefully, because there are ambiguities, uncertainties in scientific work that do not lead to immediate adjudication of some apparent discrepancies* [my emphasis].

5.   One positive outcome of this otherwise unfortunate series of events, and the wide publicity which it generated, was that it contributed to a greater alertness about research misconduct and thereby it contributed to the development of guidelines and rules set up by the Association of American Medical Colleges, the Association of American Universities, the Institute of Medicine of the National Academy of Sciences, by many universities and medical schools, and ultimately by the Department of Health and Human Services, which now allow institutions to deal more effectively with allegations of research misconduct. Some institutions, such as HMS, have adopted rules that reduce the environment that encouraged such misconduct by minimizing the importance of the quantity of publications in appointments and promotions.

6.   It is impossible to provide absolute protection from research misconduct, just as there is no way to provide absolute protection from certain crimes such as airline hijacking. However, the public has accepted the inconveniences and expenses of metal detectors and searches at airports because of the very high human and economic costs of airline hijacking, and so must the scientific community accept the inconveniences and expenses of greater vigilance and skepticism to reduce the risks of research misconduct. In fact, there has been a general "tightening" of the system during the decade since JD's misconduct first came to light. However, I doubt that the systems now generally in place could have prevented JD's misconduct, although they might have led to earlier detection in the several institutions in which JD worked.

7.   To deter misconduct, scientists must provide close supervision of trainees and must take authorship responsibilities seriously. On the

other hand, they should not overreact by endangering collegial relationships among scientific collaborators or between mentors and their trainees. Although it is certainly highly desirable to alter the motivation of scientists by deemphasizing the importance of demonstrating research accomplishments in quantitative terms and to detect misconduct earlier if it occurs, we should not delude ourselves into thinking that such measures with eliminate research misconduct. Only a rigid system requiring a researcher's superiors to supervise personally the conduct and recording of every aspect of each experiment could effectively prevent all deliberate fraud. The most creative minds will not thrive in such an environment and the most promising young people might actually be deterred from embarking on a scientific career in an atmosphere of suspicion. Second only to absolute truth, science requires an atmosphere of openness, trust, and collegiality.

REFERENCES

Harvard Medical School (1982, January 25). *Report of an Ad Hoc Advisory Committee to the Dean of the Harvard Medical School on Dishonesty in Scientific Research.* Boston: author.

National Heart, Lung and Blood Institute (1982, September). *Report of the Special Panel to Review Alleged Misconduct at Brigham and Women's Hospital/Harvard Medical School.* Bethesda: author.

Emory University (1983a, March 28). *Report of an Ad Hoc Internal Review Committee to Evaluate Research of Dr. John Darsee.* Atlanta, GA: author.

Emory University (1983b, April 14). *Report of the External Review Committee to Evaluate Research of Dr. John Darsee.* Atlanta, GA: author.

Plagiarism: The Case of Elias A. K. Alsabti

DAVID J. MILLER, PhD

BACKGROUND: PLAGIARISM

The word *plagiarism* comes from the Latin *plagiarius*, meaning "kidnapper" or "literary thief"; and it is defined as "to take (ideas, writings, etc.) from (another) and pass them off as one's own"

Having read of the case of Dr. Elias Alsabti in Broad and Wade's (1982) book, *Betrayers of the Truth*, Dr. Hersen and I had requested that one of the major protagonists in the case, Dr. Daniel Wierda, contribute a chapter outlining his impressions and reflections. Instead, Dr. Wierda offered to forward a package of information including manuscripts, professional correspondence, journal commentaries, and newspaper accoounts of the whole affair. A good part of this chapter derives from that material. I would like to express my appreciation to Dr. Wierda, as well as to Mr. Pat Condo (Assistant Director of the Monsour Medical Center Family Practice Residency Program) and Ms. Connie Gore of the *Greensburg Tribune-Review*. All three provided insightful and invaluable background information.

(*Webster's New World Dictionary*, 1988). The publication of others' ideas or writings fall on a continuum of more or less conscious intent. For example, a clear case of plagiarism exists if a college professor assigns a topic to students in a graduate seminar, reads the completed papers, refers back to the papers, lifts ideas or words from the same papers (while not acknowledging their contribution), and publishes the work solely under his own name. However, if a scientist reads a number of journal articles, combines those ideas into his or her own conceptualization, independently drafts a manuscript, and references the major contributors, a case of plagiarism would be difficult to make. Because it is one of the few instances of admitted plagiarism, the case of Dr. Elias Alsabti is an instructive illustration of the negative consequences (both personal and professional) of unethical behavior.

PRE-UNITED STATES CAREER

Elias Abdel Kuder Alsabti was born on July 31, 1954, in Basra, Iraq. Specifics of his early upbringing are unknown, but it appears that as a young man he attended Basra Medical College (1971–1974), and in 1975 (June–October) completed a summer traineeship at London's Westminster Hospital. In 1975, Alsabti first came to the attention of Iraqi academic circles, when he claimed to have invented a new test that would enable the detection of certain forms of cancer. In 1975, he was reportedly transferred to the prestigious Baghdad College of Medicine and given his own laboratory, which he named the "Al-Baath Specific Protein Reference Unit" after the political organization (i.e., the Baath party) that had enabled his transfer to Baghdad. Continuing a series of impressive accomplishments, Alsabti developed the "Bakr" method for cancer detection, which was named after the then president of Iraq, Ahmed Hassan Al-Bakr (Broad & Wade, 1982).

However, Alsabti began to have difficulties with government officials when he started charging patients fees for the cancer-screening procedure (Broad & Wade, 1982). In Iraq, which had a strict policy of socialized medicine, monetary reimbursement for a medical procedure was unacceptable. His problems evidently escalated, and early in 1977 Alsabti hid in Baghdad for 2 months. Eventually he fled to

Karbahla (Iraq), hired a guide, and went to Saudi Arabia for an unspecified period. From Saudi Arabia he proceeded to Jordan, where he was introduced to King Hussein and his brother, Crown Prince Hassan. Given the strained relations between Iraq and Jordan, this "political exile" obtained a position at the prestigious King Hussein Medical Center in the capital city of Amman, where he continued his dramatic success in cancer research (Broad, 1980a; Lawrence, 1980b).

In chapter 7, I point out that early professional mentoring can have a profound effect on a young researcher. It is interesting to note that while Alsabti was still in Basra, his mentor, Dr. Al-Sayyab, was also involved in cancer research. Like Alsabti, he had received monies from the Baath political party to pursue his scientific endeavors (Broad & Wade, 1982). Modeling for Alsabti how researchers express their appreciation, Al-Sayyab named two cancer drugs after the President (Al-Bakr) and, at the time, Vice-President (Saddam) Hussein. Unfortunately for Al- Sayyab the drugs were found to have no beneficial effect, and by 1977 he was not allowed to leave the country (Broad & Wade, 1982).

TEMPLE UNIVERSITY—PHILADELPHIA

In 1977 Alsabti met Temple University microbiologist Herman Friedman at an international meeting in Brussels. Although Iraqi-born, Alsabti told Friedman that he was a member of the Jordanian royal family and was supported by His Royal Highness Crown Prince Hassan (Broad & Wade, 1982; Lawrence, 1980b). Alsabti stated that the Jordanian government was going to send him to the United States and that he would like to work in Friedman's laboratory. True to his word, Alsabti subsequently procured a $3000-a-month allowance from the Jordanian government and a tourist visa enabling him to travel to the United States (Hopey, 1989). Unbeknown to Friedman, however, Alsabti had used his name in corresponding with the Temple administration and on September 22, 1977, Alsabti appeared unannounced at Friedman's laboratory (Broad, 1980a).

Dr. Alsabti was retained as an unpaid volunteer in Friedman's laboratory, although it soon became clear that he knew nothing at all about scientific research methods. Broad and Wade (1982) quote Friedman as stating:

> One day he came into my office and showed me a paper he was working one—a new vaccine for leukemia in Jordan. He had a hundred and fifty patients he had vaccinated and prevented from dying. The vaccine was a secret, however, and he only followed the patients for six months, whereas leukemia, of course, takes longer than six months to kill. I asked him about the method. He said the technicians did it. When I asked him some serious questions about science, it was clear that he knew nothing at all. (p.41)

Alsabti was asked to leave the laboratory and required to drop all classes. On October 31, 1977, Professor and Chairman Gerald Stockman notified the Jordanian Surgeon General, Major General David Hanania, of Alsabti's "irresponsible and nonprofessional behavior," which "forced" the university and department to withdraw all support for a visa. The department received an official apology in December 1978 (Lawrence, 1980b).

JEFFERSON MEDICAL COLLEGE— PHILADELPHIA

It is unclear how Alsabti met microbiologist E. Frederick Wheelock, but from November 1977 to April 1978 he worked in Wheelock's laboratory at Jefferson Medical College. Wheelock stated that he felt Alsabti had "not been given a fair chance at Temple. . . I tried to befriend him" (Broad, 1980a, p. 1439). While at Jefferson, Alsabti was never formally enrolled in any program but took graduate courses as a nondegree student pending verification of medical credentials.

By the time Alsabti was working at Wheelock's laboratory, he was able to present himself as an international research scholar. On an application for associate membership (which was granted) in the American College of Physicians, Alsabti stated that he had financial support from the Crown Prince of Jordan and that his goals and interests included:

[obtaining a] leukemia vaccine to continue the trials which had been strated with great success. . . searching for the cause of tumor dormancy. . . training in the field of oncology to [the] degree that permit[s] me to direct the Jordanian Cancer Society in the future. . . Ph.D. in immunology. . . [and] fellowship in clinical oncology.

He listed on his curriculum vitae that he had served an internship at King Hussein Medical Center, in Jordan, had held positions at Westminster Medical School and Queen Mary Hospital in England, and had conducted oncology research at the Specific Protein Reference Unit in Iraq and at the Royal Scientific Society of Jordan (Lawrence, 1980b, pp. 585–586).

In April 1978 two researchers in the laboratory reported to Wheelock that they had evidence Alsabti was making up research data. After a meeting with all parties involved, Wheelock found "very strong" evidence of fraud and Alsabti was asked to leave. He did not, however, depart until he had taken copies of Wheelock's unpublished manuscripts and a grant proposal. Additionally in April 1978 Alsabti failed his initial attempt to pass the Educational Commission for Foreign Medical Graduates (ECFMG) examination, which would have allowed him to sit for licensing as a physician in the United States. While professional relationships were being destroyed, Alsabti married a U.S. citizien whom he had met while at Friedman's laboratory at Temple University (Broad & Wade, 1982).

M. D. ANDERSON TUMOR HOSPITAL—HOUSTON

In September 1978 Alsabti went to R. Lee Clark (President of M. D. Anderson Tumor Hospital in Houston) with letters of introduction from the Jordanian Surgeon General. He was subsequently retained as an "unpaid volunteer lab observer" in the laboratory of Giora Mavligit. In February 1979, Alsabti asked Mavligit to review a working draft of a paper soon to be submitted for publication. However, Alsabti had mistakenly left references indicating that the manuscript had actually been written by Wheelock. Mavligit went to President Clark with the information, and Alsabti was asked to leave the hospital that same month (Lawrence, 1980b).

Soon after, Mavligit received a call from an administrator at Baylor

College of Medicine asking about Dr. Alsabti's performance at M. D. Anderson. Evidently Alsabti had applied for a residency at Baylor and had this contact not been made, Alsabti might have been admitted to Baylor's program in neurosurgery (Broad, 1980a). In February 1979 the Jordanian Crown Prince finally removed Alsabti's monetary support. Jordanian officials also stated that Alsabti had not, as claimed, worked with the Surgeon General of the Jordanian Royal Forces in producing research reports. Finally, the Jordanian embassy clarified that Alsabti was not Jordanian but had "immigrated from Iraq" (Broad, 1980a).

S. W. MEMORIAL HOSPITAL—HOUSTON

On January 8, 1979, utilizing his Iraqi citizenship, Alsabti entered the American University of the Caribbean (a "last resort [program] for would-be doctors who have been rejected by U.S. medical schools": Broad & Wade, 1982, p. 48). He also applied for U.S. citizenship based upon his Jordanian passport (Broad, 1980a). On January 23, 1980, he finally passed his ECFMG, began functioning in the family practice residency at S. W. Memorial Hospital (affiliated with the University of Texas School of Medicine), and, on May 24, 1980, obtained a medical degree from the American University of the Caribbean. While at S. W. Memorial, Alsabti told a story that was similar to tales he had related in the past—that he was born in Iraq but had suffered intense political persecution forcing him to leave the country. According to the Director of Medical Education at S. W. Memorial, "We got taken in. . . . But if other people think they wouldn't have, there're wrong" (Broad & Wade, 1982, p. 48).

January 1980 was the first time Dr. Alsabti encountered charges of plagiarism. A graduate student in Wheelock's laboratory noticed an article in the journal *Neoplasma* that looked almost identical to a section in one of Wheelock's grants (An Outbreak, 1980; Scientific Articles, 1980). On January 25, 1980, Wheelock wrote a letter to Alsabti stating, "I was very shocked to read an article. . . the great majority of that article, as you are well aware, consisted of excerpts of my own writings. . . " (Wheelock letter to Alsabti, 1980).

Wheelock demanded that Alsabti publish a retraction in *Neoplasma* and acknowledge where he had obtained the data. If an immediate response were not forthcoming, Wheelock wrote that he would publish a letter himself and take legal action. Alsabti responded on February 8, 1980, stating: "You [Wheelock] have made certain allegations which are an insult to my integrity" (quoted in Broad, 1980a, p. 1439), and he threatened his own lawsuit if Wheelock pursued the matter (Lawrence, 1980b). Wheelock did pursue the matter, however, and wrote letters to several journals: *Science, Nature, The Lancet,* and the *Journal of the American Medical Association.* On April 12, 1980, *Lancet* published an editorial that included the following statement by Wheelock:

> Two-thirds of the article consisted of an almost verbatim copy of the background section of my research grant application enttitled *Tumor Dormancy and Emergence* which had been previously submitted to the U.S. Public Health Service and subsequently funded; the remainder of the article came from early drafts of my manuscripts. The author had access to, but had not contributed to, these documents during a five-month period in my laboratory two years earlier and used these documents without my knowledge or permission. (p. 826)

Nonetheless, Alsabti now possessed a medical degree, and proceeded to apply simultaneously to two medical residency programs: one affiliated with Boston University (Carney Hospital) and the other with the University of Virginia. Alsabti signed a contract with the Virginia program on April 15 and withdrew his application from the Boston affiliate on May 1 because of unspecified "family problems" (Lawrence, 1980a, p. 735).

On April 9, 1980, an unsuspecting postdoctoral student at the Chemical Industry Institute of Toxicology (CIIT) received a letter from the Editor of the *European Journal of Cancer* (EJC). Dr. Daniel Wierda was informed that an article he had published in the *EJC* was almost identical to that published in the *Japanese Journal of Medical Science and Biology* (*JJMSB*) by Dr. E. A. K. Alsabti. Wierda drove immediately to the Duke University library and reviewed a copy of the Alsabti paper. On May 2, 1980, Wierda wrote the editor (Dr. H. J. Tagnon) of EJC and stated:

> I am appalled. To see my work pirated and published in another journal essentially graph-for-graph, word-for-word, has left me stunned. I am prepared to present whatever information is necessary to prove the

authenticity of my work and will cooperate in any way with you to resolve this matter. (Wierda letter to Tagnon, 1980)

On May 9, 1980, Tagnon wrote Wierda stating: "The manuscript was sent to referees on October 20 [1978]. The two referees were in the United States. . . . One of the two referees was dead as we discovered later and of course did not reply. The manuscript sent to him was *not* returned." It is now known that the manuscript was sent to M. D. Anderson faculty member Jeffery Gottleib, who had died 4 years earlier. Evidently Alsabti had obtained the manuscript, substituted his name (and that of two fictitious coauthors) and sent it on to the *Japanese Journal of Medical Science and Biology*, where it was published in the June 11, 1979, issue.

On May 21, 1980, Wierda wrote to the editor of the *Japanese Journal of Medical Science and Biology* requesting an "urgent response to this matter" (Plagiarism, 1980). On May 23, 1980, Wierda's coauthor Dr. Thomas Pazdernik wrote letters to the editors of *JJMSB* and the *EJC*. Finally, Leon Goldberg (President of CIIT) wrote letters to the *EJC*, the *Lancet, Nature*, the Karolinska Institute (Sweden), Institute for Scientific Information, and *Science*, stating, among other things that, "the effect of all this on Dr. Wierda has been devastating, since this is his first paper—the fruits of many years of hard work for his doctoral dissertation." On June 3, 1980, Wierda wrote Crown Prince Hassan in Amman, Jordan noting that Alsabti credited support from the Royal Scientific Society and the Crown Prince. On June 14, 1980, Wierda received a letter from the secretary to Crown Prince Hassan who assured him that "all funding to Alsabti stopped about eight months ago."

UNIVERSITY OF VIRGINIA

On June 16, 1980, in the midst of this flurry of activity, Alsabti began working in the internal medicine residency program at the Roanoke Veterans Administration Hospital (affiliated with the University of Virginia). Hospital officials soon read an article about Alsabti in *Science* (June 27), confronted him with the charges (which he denied), and that same day suspended his clinical duties and patient care privileges. In an interview in *Science* with William Broad

(1980b), Alsabti maintained that he "did not publish that [Wierda] paper . . . someone mailed it to the Japanese in my name." When asked why someone would do that, he responded, "I don't know why. There are a lot of things involved" (p. 249). He stated that he would get a lawyer and prove his innocence. Nonetheless, on July 2, 1980, he resigned from the Virginia program. Hugh Davis, Director of the Salem VA hospital where Alsabti also worked, stated prophetically: "I'm sure he'll get another residency. There's just no way in the U.S. system to keep track of him" (Broad, 1980c, p. 887).

On July 8, 1980, Wierda wrote to the managing editor of *JJMSB* requesting that the journal publish a retraction: "Your journal could set the first precedent to "righting a wrong" by publishing a retraction of the Alsabti paper. A strong reaction among the scientific community is needed since the precepts of honesty and confidentiality during the manuscript review process have been impetuously violated. . . ." On July 21, 1980, the *JJMSB* sent Wierda a copy of the retraction notice that was to be published in the next issue of the journal. Copies of the journal's investigation were also sent to the editorial boards of *Science* and *Nature*.

BOSTON UNIVERSITY

Ten days after his resignation, Alsabti reapplied to the internal medicine residency program at Boston, stating that his "family problems" had been resolved; on July 10 he began work as a house officer at Carney hospital. Lawrence (1980a, p. 735) quotes a Carney vice-president as stating, "We didn't know he had been in the Virginia Program. . . . If we had, I can assure you that we would have done some very different checking." As in Virginia, Carney administrators saw an article about Alsabti (i.e., Lawrence, 1980b) and on October 3, 1980, he was suspended. Dr. Walter Baigelman (Carney's Director of Medical Education) stated that "serious questions have been raised regarding your ethics and require that this action be taken until the situation has been investigated and clarified" (Gore, 1986). Four days later, Alsabti submitted a resignation letter listing "personal matters beyond my control" as the reason for his departure. Because no mention of was made of alleged misconduct, Carney officials declined to accept the letter. Eventually, negotiations produced a mutually acceptable resignation letter (October 8, 1980) that indicated Alsabti intended to "clarify these allegations [of plagiarism] at a later date" (*Alsabti v. Massachusetts*, 1987).

It appears that after leaving the Boston area, Alsabti may have moved to England and then to Margate, Florida. In 1981, he traveled to the state of Indiana to take his medical boards (at the time the only state that did not mandate a residency). While there, a discussion was held about his participation in a small, family practice residency in Jeanette, Pennsylvania (Gore, 1986).

MONSOUR MEDICAL CENTER

Prior to his acceptance, Alsabti forwarded a cover letter to the residency stating: "Just to expedite my application which I have not received yet, enclosed please find copies of my letters of recommendation from my training. . . . I am only 26 years old." (Pat Condo, personal communication). There were *no* publications listed on the handwritten application, although he did list the 1975 "President Albakar's [sic] Award" for the top medical student in Iraq. Included in the application materials were glowing letters from faculty on the Eupraregional Specific Protein Reference Unit (London), Westminster Hospital (London), Neuro–Diagnostic Associates of Houston, Memorial Hospital (Houston) and, Carney Hospital (Boston). Operating as a clinical physician, Alsabti completed 9 months of residency at the Monsour program (May 1, 1981, to January 29, 1982) and began applications for medical licensure.

LICENSURE AND PRIVATE PRACTICE

On April 21, 1982, he was granted a medical license in Pennsylvania. Perhaps in anticipation of future moves, Alsabti also applied for medical licensure in the states of Arkansas (May 1982), Nebraska (June 1982), and Washington (April 12, 1982). On May 13, 1982, a letter from the Department of Licensing in Washington State to the Federation of State Medical Boards of the United States contended that Dr. Alsabti had withdrawn an application for licensure after inquiry about further information on his "training and experience. . . . In the course of our background investigation, we were provided with copies of two articles which raise questions about. . . Alsabti's ethics and credentials."

It appears that in the mid-to-late 1980s even Dr. Alsabti's clinical practice was being threatened. For example, Alsabti obtained a Massachusetts license in October 1981, only to have it revoked on January 2, 1986, for allegedly misrepresenting the fact that he had been asked to resign from Carney hospital (Gore, 1986). Alsabti initially won his appeal and his license was reinstated, but it was revoked again in February 1988. In Pennsylvania Alsabti was issued a license on April 12, 1982. The license was renewed on December 10, 1986, even though Pennsylvania officials knew of the Washington State letter (Gore, 1986). Interestingly, during this period (April 27, 1983), The U.S. Department of Justice, Immigration, and Naturalization Service granted Alsabti status as a "naturalized citizen."

As a private practice physician from 1982 until 1989, Dr. Alsabti operated an office in Greensburg, Pennsylvania, was on the medical staff of Jeanette Memorial Hospital (June 1982 to June 1986) and Monsour Medical Center (1982 to 1988), and was an emergency room physician at the Ohio Valley Hospital (July 1983 to April 1989). While operating his private practice, Alsabti was apparently developing an active interest in the real estate market (Gore, personal communication, November 1990).

In September 1990, an Associated Press story indicated that Dr. Elias Alsabti was killed in an automobile accident in South Africa. Evidently he was in South Africa to observe the work of a Pretoria housing development company with intentions to start similar projects in the United States (Gore, 1990). It should be noted, however, that as of April 1991 official notification of his death from the South African governement (i.e., an official death certificate) has not been not been forthcoming, and Alsabti still possesses a valid medical license in Pennsylvania.

DISCUSSION

For department chairs, medical center administrators, and laboratory chiefs, it must be of concern that an individual such as Elias

Alsabti can produce such an impressive curriculum vitae. In the spring of 1979, he presented himself as being the author of more than 60 scientific papers, possessing M.B. and Ch.B. degrees from Basra Medical College, membership in 11 scientific societies, and as having completed postdoctoral work in England, Jordan, and the United States. Eventually, he would be able to add a medical degree, residency, licensure, and clinical experience in Texas, Massachusetts, Virginia, and Pennsylvania.

Although his curriculum vitae may appear to be distinguished, discrepancies and inconsistencies began even before Alsabti left Iraq. According to a 1989 newspaper interview, Alsabti stated: "He [Al-Bakr] was my Santa Claus. . . . He gave me everything I needed. He gave me a house and access to the presidential palace. I drove a Mercedes to class and got a nice salary. I opened up a lab and named it the Al-Baath Lab, after the ruling party (Hopey, 1989, p. A8). However, according to an 1980 *Science* article, no one in Iraq had ever heard of such a unit (Broad, 1980a). Additionally, questions have been raised about Alsabti's claims to have received medical degrees from Basra and Baghdad (Broad, 1980a). During the winter of 1990–1991, attempted communication with the Iraqi government (intended to document the educational status of Alsabti) was, understandably, nonproductive.

Regarding Alsabti's admission to plagiarizing articles, as late as 1989 he continued to maintain his innocence in the Wheelock case, stating that he "called Wheelock, and told him I wrote the proposal and wanted to publish it and send it out. . . . After it was published, Wheelock called me and said he was going to sue unless I made a retraction, but I wrote back and just said the article was my work. I make reference to Wheelock's research in the article and credit him" (Hopey, 1989, p. A8). Dr. Alsabti's denial continued although almost 10 years earlier, Wheelock was quite clear about his impressions, stating, "At the end of one [plagiarized] article, he acknowledges my help in editing one of the manuscripts. That was rubbing it in a bit" (Medical Plagiarism, 1980). As noted earlier, Alsabti maintained that someone else submitted the Wierda paper to the Japanese journal. Nonetheless, Alsabti did admit to some (unspecified) instances of plagiarism, stating as his reason: "I did it because I needed the words, needed the language, to plug my own research numbers into. . . what I did is plagiarism, but I didn't know about research methods at the time. . . I'm a good doctor, but I made a mistake, and I've been paying for it" (Hopey, 1989, p. A1).

Specific instances of plagiarism leveled against Alsabti include the following:

1. Wierda and Pazdernick (1979) versus Alsabti, Ghalib, and Salem, (1979).

2. The Wheelock grant application versus Alsabti (1978, 1979d, 1979e).

3. Alsabti and Muneir (1979) versus Pettingale and Tee (1977).

4. Alsabti (1979b) versus Pettingale, Merrett, and Tee (1977).

5. Yoshida, Okazaki, Yoshino, and Araki (1977) versus Alsabti (1979c).

6. Watkins (1973) versus Alsabti (1979a).

The *Japanese Journal of Medical Science and Biology* and *Journal of Cancer Research and Clinical Oncology* have offered retractions.

No one, other than Dr. Alsabti, will know the true motivation behind his admitted plagiarism. Alsabti maintains that he had to show the Jordanian government he was earning his keep; "I was pulling articles out of the library and plugging my own numbers into them. . . I was just doing them to massage my way with the Jordanian government" (Hopey, 1989, p. A8). Alsabti maintained that the actual data were brought with him from Iraq and Jordan. This claim is difficult to believe because comparison of several of the plagiarized papers indicate identical data, statistical analyses, and figures. Alsabti would have liked the scientific community to believe that, as a naive researcher and political exile, not familiar with the English language, he essentially used the words of others to facilitate presentation of his data. As might be expected, others see the situation differently. Mavligit stated that Alsabti was "very smart, very ambitious, and rich as hell. He does not need any money. When you've got these three things together, all you want to do is become famous" (Broad, 1980a, p 1439; Medical Plagiarism, 1980).

Evidently, Alsabti attempted to leave his research career behind. When he did so, it appeared he had learned enough clinical medicine to be an acceptable physician. According to a Carney hospital spokesperson, Alsabti was a "good intern" and performed his responsibilities in adequate fashion (Lawrence, 1980a). Additionally, Mr. Pat Condo of Monsour Medical Center stated that when he first learned of the case, he

> . . . was shocked. . . . His activity here never reflected any part of that. . . he did no research here, nor spoke of any he had participated in. . . . He could have had a fortune as a physician. . . he had great bedside manner. . . always dressed extremely neat and showed that he had a lot of money. . . they used to call him Dr. Gucci. . . but he probably envisioned himself as a great scholar and clinical professor, speaking around the world giving lectures. . . .

Indicative of how far removed was his vision from reality, as early as 1980 the deputy Jordanian ambassador to the United States stated, "If anyone can bring a legal case against him, we will be more than happy" (Broad, 1980a, p. 1438).

SUMMARY

The Alsabti case raises three specific issues for examination:

1. Hospital administrators and heads of laboratories would be wise to make personal contact with individuals whose names are submitted as references. There were many opportunities for officials to question why Alsabti was released from positions in various hospitals and universities. For example, the letters of recommendations submitted to the Monsour residency program were all somewhat dated and were submitted in a group by Alsabti. One call to Dr. Friedman in Philadelphia would have raised the question about Alsabti's scientific acumen; were it not for a fortuitous telephone call, Alsabti might have been allowed to operate as a neurosurgeon. Finally, potential employers should critically evaluate researchers who are perhaps a bit too prolific (especially when not substantially affiliated with a major laboratory). According to *Index Medicus*, Alsabti's publications record leaped from one in 1977, to 13 in 1979, and finally 19 in 1980. As Mavligit stated: "There's no doubt Alsabti knew the weaknesses of the system very well and maybe it's a lesson to all of us to be more skeptical" (Medical Plagiarism, 1980).

2. In many respects the case is an interesting demonstration of the scientific system of checks and balances. First, Alsabti worked only as volunteer or on nondegree "fellowships" requiring "outside funding" (i.e., the Jordanians paid large sums of support money). Never did Alsabti have an official academic position where his research endeavors would have been scrutinized by colleagues, Institutional Review Boards, and human subject committees. Critically, the entire case was uncovered, numerous articles written, and retractions printed within a 10-year span (a fleeting moment in the history of science).

3. It is becoming an increasingly common practice for researchers to begin a literature search through the use of a computerized indexing system. Unfortunately, a search of Medline (*Index Medicus*), Chemline (*Chemical Abstracts*), and Cancerlit (National Cancer Institute) show problematic inconsistencies in how indexing services report a journal's printed retractions. For example, Medline lists the retraction of the Alsabti, Ghalib, and Salem (1979) article in the *Japanese Journal of Medical Science and Biology*, but not the retraction in the *Journal of Cancer Research and Clinical Oncology*. Neither retraction is listed in Chemline, and Cancerlit does not include the reference.

When a scientist utilizes an index service as part of a comprehensive literature search, it is important to locate a specific citation for each printed article. For that reason, I do not recommend "purging" or completely removing all mention of fraudulent manuscripts. Rather, I would recommend an addendum or clarification in the reference of the plagiarist's article. For noncomputerized, printed indexes, I would recommend publication of an annual supplement containing all retractions.

I would also echo the recommendation that journals have a separate section for those few instances of retractions. Arnold Relman states the case very clearly: "If the manuscript in question has already been published, and the author is found guilty of fraud, the editor must be prepared to publish a prompt retraction" (Relman, 1990, p. 27). Hence, when a clear case of scientific fraud or misconduct, including plagiarism, has been established, there should be *no* editorial hesitance in printing a retraction.

REFERENCES

Alsabti, E. v. Massachusetts Board of Registration in Medicine, No. 86–37, 1987.

Alsabti, E. A. K. (1978). Tumor Dormancy: A review. *Tumor Research, 13,* 1–13.

Alsabti, E. A. K. (1979a). Lymphocyte transformation in patients with breast cancer. *Japanese Journal of Experimental Medicine, 49,* 101.

Alsabti, E. (1979b). Serum immunoglobins in breast cancer. *Journal of Surgical Oncology, 11,* 129–133.

Alsabti, E. A. K. (1979c). Serum lipids in hepatoma. *Oncology, 36,* 11.

Alsabti, E. A. K. (1979d). Tumor dormancy: A review. *Cancer Research and Clinical Oncology, 95,* 209–220.

Alsabti, E. A. K. (1979e). Tumor dormancy: A review. *Neoplasma, 26,* 351–361.

Alsabti, E. A. K., Ghalib, O. N., & Salem, M. H. (1979). Effect of platinum compounds on murine lymphocyte mitogenesis. *Japanese Journal of Medical Science and Biology, 32,* 53–65.

Alsabti, E. A. & Muneir, K. (1979). Serum proteins in breast cancer. *Japanese Journal of Experimental Medicine, 49,* 235–240.

Broad, W. J. (1980a). Would-be academician pirates papers. *Science, 208,* 1438–1440.

Broad, W. J. (1980b, July 11). Jordanian denies he pirated papers. *Science,* **209,** 249.

Broad, W. J. (1980c, August 22). Jordanian accused of plagiarism quits job. *Science, 209,* 886–887.

Broad, W. J., & Wade, N. (1982). *Betrayers of the truth.* New York: Touchstone.

Gore, C. (1986, November 24). Local doctor facing license review hearing, *Greensburg Tribune-Review,* pp. A4, A7.

Gore, C. (1990, September 30). Former area doctor killed in S. Africa. *Greensburg Tribune-Review.*

Hopey, D. (1989, March 5). 10 years later, plagiarism may cost doctor his license in state. *The Pittsburgh Press,* pp. A1, A8.

Lawrence, S. V. (1980a). Alsabti resigns again. *Forum on Medicine,* 735.

Lawrence, S. V. (1980b). "Let no one else's work evade your eyes. . . ". *Forum on Medicine,* 582–587.

Medical plagiarism. (1980, June 27). *Houston Post.*

An outbreak of piracy in the literature. (1980). *Nature, 285*, 429–430.

Plagiarism strikes again. (1980, July 31). *Nature, 286*, 433.

Pettingale, K. W., Merrett, T. G., & Tee, D. E. H. (1977). Prognostic value of serum levels of immunoglobins (IgG, IgA, IgM, and IgE) in breast cancer: A preliminary study. *British Journal of Cancer, 36*, 550–557.

Pettingale, K. W., & Tee, D. E. H. (1977). Serum protein changes in breast cancer: A prospective study. *Journal of Clinical Pathology, 30*, 1048–1052.

Relman, A. S. (1990). Publishing biomedical research: Roles and responsibilities. *Hastings Center Report, 20*, 23–27.

Scientific articles believed pirated. (1980, June 28). *Richmond Times-Dispatch.*

Special Correspondent. (1980, July 5). Must plagiarism survive? *British Medical Journal*, 41–42.

Watkins, S. M. (1973). The effects of surgery on lymphocyte transformation in patients with breast cancer. *Clinical and Experimental Immunology, 14*, 69.

Webster's New World Dictionary (3rd College Ed.). (1988). New York: Simon & Schuster.

Wheelock, E. F. (1980). Plagiarism and freedom of information laws. *Lancet, 1*, 826.

Wierda, D., & Pazdernick, T. L. (1979). Suppression of spleen lymphocytes mitogenesis in mice injected with platinum compounds. *European Journal of Cancer, 15*, 1013–1023.

Yoshida, T., Okazaki, N., Yoshino, M., & Araki, E. (1977). Diagnostic evaluation of serum lipids in patients with hepatocellular carcinoma. *Japanese Journal of Clinical Oncology, 7*, 15–20.

Scientific Fraud or False Accusations? The Case of Cyril Burt

ARTHUR R. JENSEN, PhD

OVERVIEW

The case of Sir Cyril Burt is probably the most bizarre episode in the entire history of academic psychology. This is due to a unique combination of elements—the socially touchy subject of Burt's major research; his genuinely outstanding accomplishments; his mysteriously complex character; and finally, some years after his death, the damaging accusations leveled against him and the extreme and strangely virulent vilification of his reputation that ensued. Burt's posthumous worldwide notoriety surely exceeds the considerable fame and acclaim he enjoyed during his long and immensely distinguished career.

What became known as the "Burt scandal" surfaced in 1976, five years after his death. The mass media broadcast blatant accusations of scientific fraud. In his famous study of the IQs of 53 pairs of identical twins reared apart, Burt was accused faking data and fabricating both research assistants and coauthors to lend it authenticity.

This sensational attack on Burt seemed flimsy to most professionals who knew the available facts. The claims appeared to be nothing more than highly speculative inferences from circumstantial evidence. The attackers aimed to discredit Cyril Burt, but the main thrust of their effort was to discredit this theory, as well as the body of research that supports it. Discrediting Burt and what he stood for was welcome news to the egalitarians and environmentalists who abhored his theory that genetic factors are strongly involved in human intelligence.

Burt was not without his supporters. A number of scholars, mainly former associates, rose to his defense by writing articles and letters to the newspapers, as well as making TV appearances. The controversy remained in this unsteady state of suspension for 3 years.

Burt's guilt was virtually clinched when Britain's leading and most highly respected historian of psychology, Leslie Hearnshaw (1979), published what appeared to be a carefully researched and impartial biography of Burt. The biographer had exclusive access to Burt's private correspondence and diaries, which no one else had yet seen. Thus, the generally magnificent biography (except for a few critical exceptions which I will discuss later) was almost universally accepted as the last word on the subject and even converted most of Burt's earlier supporters. The devastation of Burt's once exalted reputation was a gleeful triumph to his detractors and a tragedy to his admirers. So be it. With sighs of relief, the matter appeared settled at last.

Or so most of us thought.

Then, surprise! Recently, the whole matter has been exhumed and scrutinized anew, with an exceptional thoroughness not previously seen in the case. The plot thickens terribly. The new investigations now take a bewildering twist that turns the tables on the small band of Burt's original accusers and his distinguished biographer. This current state of affairs should be a source of chagrin to all those, including myself, who had so completely abandoned our doubts and accepted as final the guilty verdict of Burt's biographer, on the basis of simple faith in his scholarship and objectivity, without ourselves having checked into all of the purportedly damning evidence with sufficient thoroughness.

This shocking realization was brought home by the assiduous investigative efforts of two scholars responsible for reopening the case. They are two British professors, Robert B. Joynson (1989) and Ronald Fletcher (1991), in psychology and sociology, respectively. Neither one knew Burt personally nor ever had any previous connection with any aspect of Burt's research or the "IQ controversy." Joynson's involvement resulted from a particular accusation in Hearnshaw's (1979) biography having to do with Burt's role in the development of factor analysis, a mathematical technique that became a major methodology in quantitative and statistical psychology. Fletcher, amazed at the sensationalism of the Burt exposé in the popular media and the odium so flagrantly heaped on Burt in the absence of any official investigation, suspected that a grave injustice had been perpetrated. It seemed essential to take a close look at the purported evidence for the claimed malfeasance. The two investigators, working independently, devoted several years to carrying out what appears to be extraordinarily meticulous detective work on the Burt affair. Each has published a book reporting the results of their examination of the charges and the evidence. Though both critically question every accusation and sift meticulously through evidence, their accounts differ markedly in organization and style. With regard to the main charges, the two authors reach the same conclusion: *Not proven.*

What effect on scholarly opinion this recent massive defense of Burt might have remains uncertain and depends on whether the defense can be convincingly and honestly refuted. So far, no effective refutation of any points in the case for the defense has appeared. If that should remain so, it clearly gives Burt the benefit of the legal dictum—"innocent until *proven* guilty"—which of course, only means "proven beyond reasonable doubt."

Many, I imagine, will feel that these recent investigations have at least established a reasonable doubt that Burt committed fraud. But perhaps I have become too wary in this controversy to bet on an eventual resolution. The verdict of history, as well as public opinion and private opinion, are not bound by the rules of a court of law. Even if there remains room for reasonable and irresolvable doubt, the final outcome will likely be a hung jury—split three ways. There will be those who deliberately remain agnostic and others for whom some prejudice, probably more than any other factor, will determine their preference to give the benefit of the doubt either to Burt or to his detractors.

Before getting into the details of this perplexing case, it is important first to know just who Burt was, what he did as a researcher, and what he was like personally. Certain features of his personality, and especially his area of research, prepared the fertile ground for the "Burt scandal" to sprout and flourish.

WHO WAS BURT?

Sir Cyril Lodovic Burt (1883–1971) was unquestionably one of the dominant figures in the history of British psychology. He was the first British psychologist to be knighted (a distinction bestowed on only two other psychologists to date). In his lifetime, his eminence was rivaled by few contemporaries—exceptions include Charles Spearman, Britain's greatest psychologist, and at some distance perhaps William McDougall, Sir Frederick Bartlett, and Sir Godfrey Thomson. Most would agree that Burt had all the appearance of a "great man." His intellectual brilliance and scholarly industry were legendary, and in terms of academic accomplishments and influence, degrees, honors, awards, and the like, he was a towering figure.

After graduating from Oxford University, where he studied classics, mathematics, physiology, and psychology, Burt worked for 4 years as an assistant to the celebrated neurophysiologist Sir Charles Sherrington at Liverpool University. Following a stint as a lecturer in experimental psychology at Cambridge, he was appointed in 1913 as psychologist to the London County Council. This position put Burt in charge of psychological research and applied psychology, including the development of mental and scholastic tests, for the entire London school system. In this setting he became one of the world's leading educational psychologists and psychometricians, developing new tests, conducting surveys, founding child guidance clinics and a special school for the handicapped, and pioneering research on juvenile delinquency and mental retardation. Some of these studies he reported in beautifully written books that became classics in their field: *The Young Deliquent* (1925), *The Subnormal Mind* (1935), and *The Backward Child* (1937).

During much of the period that Burt held his appointment with the London County Council, he also occupied the chair in educational psychology at the University of London. When Charles Spearman, one of the great pioneers of mental testing, retired in 1932 as professor (and head) of the Department of Psychology in University College, London, Burt inherited his position, probably the most influential in British psychology.

Burt retired in 1950 at the age of 68. The last 20 years of his life were spent in a rather reclusive life-style, living in a large London flat with a secretary-housekeeper, editing journals and writing books and articles. He was remarkably prolific even in his old age. Following his retirement, he published more than 200 articles and reviews. And those were only the items published under his *own* name. In addition, as his most notable eccentricity, he wrote a considerable number of articles, mostly book reviews (it remains uncertain just how many), under various pseudonyms or initials of unidentifiable names. He worked steadily almost until the day he died, at the age of 88.

Burt published in the areas of general psychology, the history of psychology, philosophical psychology and methodology, intelligence, mental retardation, giftedness, educational psychology, parapsychology, and the psychology of typography. But the two areas of research for which he was best known, and which he himself regarded as the fields of his most important scientific contributions, were *factor analysis* and the *genetics of intelligence*, fields in which his excellent mathematical aptitude could be used to great advantage.

In both of these fields, Burt was undeniably an outstanding pioneer. This is true despite the damaging peculiarities and faults found in some of his articles on the IQ correlations of twins and other kinships. There is little question that in his grasp of the then new theories and methodology of quantitative genetics being developed by geneticists such as Sir Ronald Fisher, J. B. S. Haldane, and Kenneth Mather, Burt was well ahead of all of his contemporaries in the behavioral and social sciences. He expertly adapted these new developments in quantitative genetics to the study of human behavioral traits. Kinship correlations are the essential data for quantitative genetic analysis, and beginning quite early in his career, while still working in the London schools, Burt started collecting IQs and scholastic achievement scores on twins and various other kinshps. Between the years

1943 and 1966 (and a posthumously published article in 1972) he published many theoretical and empirical studies dealing with the inheritance of intelligence.

It was particularly this *genetic* aspect of Burt's psychometric studies of individual differences that seemed to have such controversial educational and social implications. Egalitarian ideologues tended to view the so-called nature–nurture question as a political issue, rather than as a scientific one, and so the potential controversy extended to a much larger arena than just the field of behavioral genetics.

Burt himself, however, was not at all a political animal. He seldom expressed any interest in politics, never joined any political party, and those who knew him personally only surmised he was a liberal of the old-fashioned kind, just slightly "left of center." Apparently no one who ever knew him thought him to have Conservative sympathies, and it is noteworthy that his knighthood was awarded by Britain's Labour party (Hearnshaw, 1979, pp. 126–127).

Burt's personality is a much more puzzling matter. I knew Burt personally and enjoyed numerous visits with him in the last 2 years of his life, which I have detailed elsewhere (Jensen, 1983) in a most interesting collection of reminiscences about Burt by a number of people who knew him personally, many better than I did. My direct impressions need no revision in light of the later controversey. They were summed up in my obituary on Burt (Jensen, 1972), as follows:

> What sort of man was Burt personally? Undoubtedly he had strong views and opinions, and at times he could be quite combative intellec- tually in defending them. He was devastating in debate. One would be rather hard put to characterize Sir Cyril, even in his late eighties, as "mild" or as a "grand old man." Nor would he have liked such an image. He had a keenly critical disposition and was quick to point out one's intellectual lapses and to pursue an argument relentlessly. Those who disagreed with him were not let off easily. I was privileged to have become quite well acquainted with Sir Cyril in his later years and to have had many visits and conversations with him. He was most gener- ous. The overall picture that Sir Cyril leaves in one's memory, after corresponding with him, seeing him, and conversing with him is very clear indeed. Everything about the man—his fine, sturdy appearance, his aura of vitality, his urbane manner, his unflagging enthusiasm for research, analysis, and criticism; even such a small detail as his firm, meticulous handwriting; and, of course, especially his notably sharp

intellect and vast erudition—all together leave a total impression of immense quality, of a born nobleman (p. 117)

But it was obvious to Burt that I was an admirer, and probably his relationship to me, always friendly and generous, was not entirely typical of his dealings with individuals who new him as a faculty colleague or as a teacher. Opinions of Burt vary widely among this group, ranging from the highest esteem to bitter denigration, both at times coming even from the same observer. There are only three characteristics about which everyone agrees: Burt's exceptional intellectual brilliance, his extraordinary general erudition, and his untiring industry.

The less favorable impressions of Burt registered by a few of his former students, colleagues, and acquaintances mention his egocentrism and personal vanity, his autocratic manner in running his department, his insistence on getting his own way, and his obsessive need to have the last word in any argument. Also, as a noted colleague Philip E. Vernon wrote, "It seemed difficult for him to allow his past students or followers to branch out and publish contributions which went beyond his views" (Vernon, 1972, p. 6). Vernon (1987) also wrote, "Although Burt gave immense amounts of help to students and others, he could not brook any opposition to his views, and often showed paranoic tendencies in his relations with colleagues and critics" (p. 159). In connection with Vernon's latter statement, it is noteworthy that such psychiatrically tinged opinions were never in evidence, at least in print, until *after* the accusation of fraud had been endorsed by Burt's biographer (Hearnshaw, 1979), who himself led the way by heavily "psychologizing" his explanation of Burt's purported crimes.

Burt's most famous student, Professor Hans J. Eysenck, even entitled one of his many articles on Burt as "Polymath and Psychopath" (Eysenck, 1983). However, I do recall conversations with Eysenck, even many years before Burt's death, in which he referred to Burt as being "very neurotic" and described some of Burt's eccentricities and peculiar deviousness in personal relationships. I had no reason ever to question these remarks. They never seemed vindictive but evinced only disappointment or amusement. Eysenck has always held the same views as Burt's concerning the nature of intelligence and its heritability; he strongly defended Burt at the first accusation of fraud

(Eysenck, 1977); and he even dedicated one of his books to Burt (as did at least four other authors that I know of, including myself). Space limitation here does not permit the details needed adequately to present Eysenck's perception of what could be called the eccentric side of Burt's personality, about which Eysenck has written more perhaps than anyone except Burt's biographer (Eysenck, 1980a, 1980b, 1982, 1983, 1989). The most damaging example, in my opinion, is Eysenck's (1983) account of how Burt wrote the first draft of a critical review of an important book by Leon Thurstone, and in this review Burt's own method of factor analysis was shown to give a result that contradicted Thurstone's method applied to the same data—a point of considerable theoretical dispute at that time. Eysenck, as a student research assistant to Burt, had performed the laborious factor analysis of Thurstone's data at Burt's request, and for doing so was promised coauthorship. But when the review was finally published, Eysenck's name surprisingly appeared as the sole author (Eysenck, 1939). Burt had made his points and escaped any personal risk of a backlash from Thurstone.

Eysenck is not entirely alone in his perception of "abnormalities" in Burt's personality, and although such impressions have now become a part of the total picture, it should also be emphasized that some of Burt's closest acquaintances have never reported anything like these unfavorable characterizations (see, e.g., Association of Educatioal Psychologists, 1983). Moreover, the severely critical "cross-examination" of Eysenck regarding his accounts of Burt's alleged peccadillos by both Joynson (1989, Ch. 10) and Fletcher (1991, Ch. 6) should give the reader pause. They are probably correct in arguing that this kind of personal testimony and hearsay evidence would not be admissible in a court of law. I can conclude only by stressing this point: A composite of all of the personal recollections of Burt's characteristics I have read or encountered in conversations with those who knew him, along with my own direct impressions of him, indeed presents a conflicting and perplexing picture.

PUZZLING PECULIARITIES IN BURT'S HERITABILITY STUDIES

Perhaps the only objective means for evaluating Burt is to judge him by the published work he left behind. His strictly theoretical contributions on factor analysis and on the polygenic theory of intelligence are unquestionably brilliant and important. But his empirical research is a rather different story, leading to questions and doubts. The contrast between Burt's impressive theoretical and quantitative sophistication and the apparently lesser care with which he reported crucial empirical data, with its overly sparing and even rather slipshod manner of presentation, might even suggest that Burt lacked essential qualities of an experimental scientist.

Within a few days after the news of Burt's death in 1971, I wrote to Miss Gretl Archer, who was Burt's private secretary for over 20 years, to request that she preserve the two or three tea crates of old raw data that Burt had once told me he still possessed. I told Miss Archer that I would travel to London the following summer to go through this material. I supposed they probably included IQ test data on twins, in which I had an interest and thought could be used in certain newer kinds of genetic analysis that Burt had not applied. Miss Archer replied that all of these data had been destroyed within days after Burt's death, on the advice of Dr. Liam Hudson, Professor of Educational Psychology in Edinburgh University. He had come to Burt's flat soon after the announcement of Burt's death. Miss Archer, distraught and anxious to vacate Burt's large and expensive flat in Hampstead, had already arranged for the disposition of Burt's library and correspondence files (which were turned over to his biographer, Hearnshaw), but she expressed concern to Hudson about what to do with these boxes of old data. Hudson looked over their contents and advised that she burn them, as being no longer of any value. Miss Archer said she believed the boxes included the data on twins, and she later expressed regret that she had acted on Hudson's advice. (The account I received from Miss Archer of this event was completely corroborated by Hudson himself, in a telephone interview with *Science* staff writer Nicholas Wade, 1976.)

I was flabbergasted when I received this news of the destruction of whatever had still existed of Burt's data. I was especially flabbergasted because it was obvious that, although Miss Archer knew of Hudson only by name and that he was a professor at Edinburgh, she had no idea that he was one of Burt's most ardent antihereditarian opponents. I had met Hudson in 1970 at Cambridge University in a debate for which he had been selected by the sponsors to oppose my position (and Burt's) regarding the heritability of intelligence. While having breakfast with Hudson the morning before the debate, I brought up the subject of Burt (who was alive and well at that time), and I was struck by Hudson's unkind remarks about Burt, which expressed a strong, emotionally toned antipathy toward Burt's views. (Hudson had never met Burt personally.) Hudson later published a book, *The Cult of the Fact* (1972), in which the "bad guys" are hereditarians, including Galton, Spearman, Burt, Eysenck, and me. Still later, Hudson wrote the Foreword to the Penguin edition of Leon Kamin's (1974) book attacking Burt and the whole hereditarian position on IQ. Both Hudson's rush to Burt's flat right after his death and his advice to Burt's secretary-housekeeper to burn the stored data seem stranger than fiction. Surely, it must be one of the most bizarre events in the whole Burt affair.

Although Burt's data were no longer available for new analysis, I thought I could still perform a service to the field of behavior genetics by publishing an article that systematically assembled all of the kinship correlations Burt had ever reported in his various publications in different journals. So in the summer of 1972 following Burt's death, I visited Miss Archer, who allowed me to go through Burt's reprint files in search of any of his articles reporting kinship studies that I did not possess.

From all of Burt's journal articles that deal with the heritability of IQ, I systematically tabulated every type of kinship correlation or other statistic (e.g., monozygotic twins reared apart [MZA] or reared together [MZT], dizygotic twins, siblings, parent–child, etc.) for every type of variable on which Burt had obtained measurements (e.g., IQ—both group and individual tests, achievement in various scholastic subjects, and various physical measurements), and presented them in a set of nine large tables (in Jensen, 1974). Seeing all of the Kinship correlations systematically laid out in this way, in contrast to encountering them scattered throughout a number of different journal articles, I was immediately struck by numerous peculiarities in the pattern of correlations for the various kinships.

The most conspicuous peculiarity was the exact repetition of the same correlation coefficients from one report to the next, despite changing sample size. As one example, take what is probably the most informative of all kinship correlations for genetic inference, namely, MZ twins reared apart (MZA). Burt published several articles reporting such MZA correlations for IQ, as follows (for detailed references to this, see Jensen [1974] and Joynson [1989, Ch. 6]):

Year	N	Correlation
1943	15	.77
1955	21	.771
1956	?	.7706
1958	?	.771
1966	53	.771

Similar repetitions of identical correlations were also reported for other kinships, for measurements of general intelligence, scholastic achievement, and physical characteristics. I counted about 20 such "invariant" correlations and other numerical anomalies in all of the tables of Burt's kinship statistics. It is impossible here to describe all these in any detail, but this has been done elsewhere (Jensen, 1974, 1978) and, even more thoroughly and analytically, by Joynson (1989, Ch. 6). The upshot of these examinations of Burt's figures can be summarized in a series of points:

1. Very few of the repetitions among all of the various kinship correlations represent anything other than carrying over of the correlations reported in one article to a subsequent article. For example, in the MZA correlations listed above, Burt's 1956 and 1958 articles do not present new correlations; in fact, Burt's whole 1958 table of kinship correlations is simply an exact reproduction of the correlation table given in the 1955 article, except that in 1958 Burt did not report the Ns (15, 21, 53, respectively). The question, then, is whether three such close correlations could be pure coincidence or are so highly improbable as to prove that they must be fraudulent.

First, it is important to note that these correlations are not based on entirely independent samples. Burt cumulated his kinship data from one study to the next, and his calculations of the kinship correlations were based on the cumulated data. Hence the variation among the correlation coefficients obtained at later points in the cumulation would be expected to be considerably less than would be expected statistically for correlations based on completely independent samples.

Second, as I have noted elsewhere (Jensen, 1974, pp. 12, 14), two other studies of MZA, which were entirely independent of Burt's studies (and of one another), both report MZA correlations for IQ of precisely .77.

Third, the most recent study of MZA, by Thomas Bouchard and his associates at the University of Minnesota, which was completely independent of all the earlier studies, found a correlation of .78 on the Raven–Mill–Hill IQ and a correlation of .78 on the general intelligence factor of a battery of cognitive tests (Bouchard, Lykken, McGue, Segal, & Tellegen, 1990). It is thus a reasonable statistical inference that the true correlation of MZA for general intelligence most probably falls between .75 and .80, as does Burt's .77. Then consider also that the standard error of the observed correlation coefficient decreases as the true (or population) correlation approaches 1 (on a scale of 0 to 1). So, with a population correlation probably close to .77, the obtained sample correlations would most likely fall within a quite restricted range, as indeed was shown to be the case for three entirely independent studies of unquestioned authenticity. In short, the consistency of Burt's MZA correlations does not seem so improbable as to imply fraud.

2. It also seems unlikely that anyone with Burt's statistical sophistication who intended to fake his results would repeat the same exact correlations across samples of increasing size. It is hard to imagine that even the stuipidest undergraduate in Statistics 1A would do that.

3. Many of the peculiarities in Burt's tables are obviously errors in copying figures, consisting of reversals of digits or even putting certain numbers in the wrong column. These irregularities seem to be related to Burt's age at the time of writing the articles, most of them after he was 75 years old. They are obviously due to failures in copying from one table to another, or in not catching printing errors in the page proofs. (Burt himself later corrected some of these errors in the reprints of his articles.) For example, between 1955 and 1966 the N for DZ twins changed from 172 to 127, even though the correlations (for height and weight) remained unchanged. The 172 is obviously just a miscopying of 127, not an attempt to put something over on his readers. The same types of copying errors are found in Burt's presentation of a correlation table from the famous twin study by Newman, Freeman, and Holzinger (1937); and certainly there would be no point in his faking *their* results, which could be readily checked in their monograph (details in Jensen, 1974, Table II, p. 11).

In brief, I believe there are simply no irregularities in any of Burt's presentation of his results that are not most reasonably viewed as just careless errors. The sparseness of reporting details of testing procedures, precisely which tests were used, the ages of the subjects, and other statistics that would be useful information to other investigators are not much out of keeping with the general style of reporting studies in British journals at that time. Burt's main articles on the heritability of IQ were not published in the *British Journal of Statistical Psychology*, of which he was the founder and editor, but in other leading journals of the British Psychological Society, and they obviously passed muster with the journal editors and referees at that time. However, they would in some cases be unacceptable by present-day standards in the psychometric and behavior genetics literature.

4. The IQ scores of the 53 pairs of MZA, which Burt made available to at least five other researchers[1] who requested these data, have undergone detailed statistical comparisons with the data of all three of the other main MZA studies ever reported in the literature. Burt's raw IQ data are not at all out of line. The distribution of intrapair differences in Burt's twin sample does not show any statistically significant differences from the samples in the other studies with respect to any distribution parameters (e.g., mean, standard deviation, skewness, or kurtosis) (Jensen, 1974, pp. 15–16). Newton Morton, a leading American geneticist, made a detailed comparison between Burt's kinship correlations and all of the parallel studies done by American researchers, and he found the slight differences between the two sets of results to be statistically nonsignificant. He wrote, "Whatever errors may have crept into his [i.e., Burt's] material, they do not appear to be systematic" (cited in Jensen, 1977, p. 471–472). Also, Joynson (1989, p. 159) notes that in Burt's successive articles the pattern of the various MZ and DZ twin and sibling correlations tends to change in ways that would actually *decrease* the heritability coefficient, hence strengthening environmental causation of IQ differences—a most unlikely ploy indeed if Burt were faking results to bolster an hereditarian argument.

5. Because of the prima facie inaccuracies and ambiguities in Burt's heritability studies, now compounded with unresolvable doubts about his data's authenticity, behavioral geneticists have prop-

[1]Burt sent the IQ and SES data on his MZ twins reared apart to Professors L. Erlenmeyer-Kimling, Chistopher Jencks (see Joynson, 1989, p. 193). Sandra Scarr, William Shockley, and John J. Werth (copies of the latter three persons' correspondence with Burt, including his replies, are in my possession).

erly dismissed Burt's figures from further consideration. Since at least 1980 Burt's correlations have been intentionally omitted from literature reviews, summaries, meta-analyses, or any heritability estimates based on combined data from past studies.

Scientifically, the dismissal of Burt's empirical legacy was not much of a substantive loss, because by that time many other independent studies of the heritability of intelligence already existed, and large-scale studies were well underway to replicate Burt's theoretically most crucial kinship correlations, such as those for MZA. The "Burt affair" per se had become a matter only of historical and biographical interest, with no strictly scientific consequences for the progress of behavior genetics. But Burt's place in the history of psychology would be quite different if his conclusions about the heritability of intelligence had not turned out to be essentially correct. In that event it seems most unlikely that two decades after his death scholars would be concerned to rehabilitate his image, not as a scientific issue, but as the righting of an injustice for the historical record.

ACCUSATIONS OF FRAUD

The first public accusation of outright fraud appeared on October 24, 1976, in the London *Sunday Times*, under the striking headline: "Crucial Data Was Faked by Eminent Psychologist," written by Oliver Gillie (1976a), the *Times*'s medical correspondent. Within days the story was repeated in the mass media around the world. Gillie followed with other sensational articles under headlines such as "the great IQ fraud" and "the scandal and the cover-up," and a style replete with vilification—"outright fraud," "fraudster," "plagiarist of long standing."

These charges were not based on anything new involving Burt's data, the peculiarities of which had already been pointed out two years earlier. They rested on the claim that Gillie had been unable either to locate in person or to find any trace of two women— Margaret Howard and J. Conway—who were credited with assisting Burt in his research on twins. Howard was a coauthor of one of Burt's most important articles on twins and Conway was named as the sole author of an article that was actually written by Burt himself, according to his secretary. These two women could not be traced or even identified with certainty by anyone available for questioning who had been associated with Burt. The "missing ladies," as Gillie called them, gave him licence to claim that Burt's data were, as he put it, "faked."

There is a sidelight to this story that has not yet been recorded anywhere. So, as an eyewitness, I think I should tell it. Although it may seem trivial, I think it is a clue to understanding much of what actually followed. It should be prefaced by two items of information: (1) Shortly before his *Sunday Times* exposé on Burt, Gillie (1976b) published a popular book that took a strongly environmentalist stance and was antagonistic toward the idea of inherited differences in mental qualities; (2) Gillie credited Professor Jack Tizard (since deceased, but then a psychologist in London University's Institute of Education) with helping him search for the "missing ladies." Tizard, although he had scarcely known Burt personally, became an active participant in the attack on Burt, giving Gillie information and advice on how to go about it (see Joynson, 1989, pp. 283–288).

I was well acquainted with Tizard, having spent two years (1956–1958) in London in the same psychology department where Tizard was at that time. In frequent lunchtime conversations with him, I found him intensely political and, like so many other Communist[2] intellectuals of that period, a "passionate egalitarian," to use his wife's characterization (as quoted by Joynson, 1989, p. 296). He was quite outspokenly antihereditarian and anti-Burtian. During the following years, I saw Tizard occasionally on my visits to London.

On one such occasion, well before Gillie's exposé of Burt, I told Tizard about the recent publication of my 1974 summation of Burt's kinship data and asked him if he knew anything about Burt's assistants, Howard and Conway. I had already sought this information from several of Burt's former associates, because I thought it would be interesting to talk with these women who were credited with collecting some of Burt's data on twins. When I mentioned to Tizard that I had not yet come across anyone who knew anything about these women, except for having seen their names in Burt's articles, his eyes veritably lit up. He excitedly said something to the effect that perhaps these women never existed at all and were just pure figments, and he

[2]According to an interview with Tizard that appeared in the *APA Monitor*, Tizard was a member of the Communist party (Evans, 1977, p. 4).

loudly clapped his hands. His exclamation still rings vividly in my memory: "Wouldn't it be great if it could be shown that Burt was really just an old fraud!" At that moment I thought, how perfectly his reaction epitomized wishful thinking about smashing Burt and ipso facto the whole hereditarian position.

Then, sure enough, the day after Gillie's sensational charges of fraud in the *Sunday Times*, there appeared in *The Times* (October 25, 1976) an interview with Tizard, headed "Theories of IQ pioneer 'completely discredited'." It began: "The theory of Sir Cyril Burt. . . that man's intelligence is largely caused by heredity was now completely discredited, Professor Jack Tizard, Professor of Child Development at London University, said yesterday. . . . Professor Tizard said the discrediting of Burt's work cast doubt on his whole line of inquiry," (Devlin, 1976).

This telling episode suggests that the main steam behind the attack on Burt may have been the fervent wish of environmentalists to discredit the theory of the polygenic inheritance of mental ability and all other behavioral traits of obvious personal, educational, and social importance. Such indeed was the leitmotiv in the popular press and TV, both in England and America. (It even predominates in accounts of Burt in some psychology textbooks.) Because ideological propaganda depends not on facts, but on images, impressions, and prejudices, the anti- Burt campaign naturally avoided the fact that Burt's research was in line with the consensus of other expert studies on the heritability of IQ (Bouchard et al., 1990; Plomin, 1987, 1990). This key phenomenon was perfectly capsulized by Raymond Cattell (personal communication, 1979; also see Cattell, 1980): "The mass media conveyed to a large public that any inheritance of intelligence was a myth, and Burt became the effigy of behavior genetics, in whose burning all claims for genetic inequalities and differences hopefully went up in smoke."

HEARNSHAW'S BIOGRAPHY: A CRUCIAL VERDICT

When the scandal broke in the media, it was already known in psychological circles that Professor Leslie Hearnshaw (1907–1991) had been working for several years on what would become the "official" biography of Burt. Because of Hearnshaw's well-recognized scholarly credentials as an historian of psychology, and the fact that he had no prior involvement in the "IQ controversy" or in any other aspect of Burt's activity, his objectivity and credibility in the Burt case were unblemished. Also, he had delivered a beautiful eulogy at Burt's memorial service and was commissioned to write the biography by Burt's sister, who made available all of Burt's diaries and correspondence. It was everyone's reasonable expectation that Hearnshaw's forthcoming biography of Burt would become generally regarded as the authoritative last word on the subject, providing "the whole truth and nothing but the truth" in so far as it could be ascertained from the available evidence.

Especially after Gillie's sensational charges against Burt, Hearnshaw's biography was eagerly awaited. And there was a sense of urgency, either for damage control or to clinch the case authoritatively. Unfortunately, the full-blown scandal exposed by Tizard and Gillie fell on Hearnshaw while he was already in the late stage of his writing. It was mandatory, of course, for his biography to deal with it fully.

Several of Burt's detractors grabbed this opportunity and prevailed on Hearnshaw personally, offering further accusations that had not previously come to light. The most curiously assiduous in this effort were two psychologists at Hull University, Alan and Ann Clarke (husband and wife), who had both earned their PhDs under Burt back in 1950. They claimed (see Joynson, 1989, pp. 244–245) that Burt had written and published articles under *their* names, based on their own doctoral dissertations, and that he had also "slanted" their conclusions to his own purpose—an accusation that further built up doubts of Burt's integrity and created an image of him as being (to use the Clarkes' own words) "unscrupulous," a "rogue," "con man," "confidence trickster," and "fraud." (see Fletcher, 1987, 1991). The Clarkes repeated this charge many times in articles and on the BBC radio. Hearnshaw seemingly accepted this defamatory charge at face value, without verifying it, and incorporated it wholesale into his biography (p. 148) as a flagrant example of Burt's devious character.

Burt's detractors were obviously successful in impressing Hearnshaw of Burt's guilt, and "Hearnshaw, once convinced, wrote a prosecution brief,'' as Cronbach (1979, p. 1393) concluded in his review of Hearnshaw's book. Joynson (1989) also is quotable on this point:

> Thus we reach the striking conclusion that none of the main charges that Hearnshaw brought against Burt had actually originated in his own research. In every case, the suspicion first came from others. It is an instructive reflection that, if Hearnshaw had been left in peace to complete his work in his own time and his own way, it is unlikely that he would ever have accused Burt of dishonesty at all. (p. 312)

When Hearnshaw's massive and impressively well-written biography was published in 1979, his conclusions of guilt on several counts became widely accepted, even by most of Burt's former defenders. The Council of the British Psychological Society (BPS) endorsed Hearnshaw's conclusions and officially declared Burt's guilt in a booklet entitled *A Balance Sheet on Burt* (Beloff, 1980). The "balance sheet,'' however, is clearly anything *but* balanced. Both Tizard and Alan Clarke were members of the BPS Council when it planned for the official pronouncement on Burt (Joynson, 1989, pp. 316–321). And if ever there was a kangaroo court, this was it. Among the seven presenters in the *Balance Sheet* were Hearnshaw, Gillie, Ann Clarke, and Alan Clarke. They alone constituted the prosecutor, judge, and jury. As expected, they all roundly condemned Burt, while the remaining three contributors, who had never visibly done any research into the Burt affair, simply acquiesced in the official pronouncement and wrote only in general terms on research methodology and scientific fraud. As far as is known, there was no attempt to question the evidence claimed to support any of the several charges against Burt.

Why were so many so convinced by Hearnshaw's book? I myself had reviewed the manuscript for the publisher and praised it highly. Its cool-headed, judicious style evinced absolutely none of the rancor or antihereditarian rhetoric typical of Burt's detractors. What seemed to be the crucial evidence in Hearnshaw's exclusive possession were Burt's diaries and correspondence. The diaries covered the period (1953–1960) in Burt's career that seemed most in question regarding the acquisition of new twin data. Hearnshaw gives the impression that the diaries were quite complete and detailed, recording even such insigificant things as Burt's having tea with a friend, taking a walk, or getting a haircut. Surely anyone would think that anything as exciting and important and rare as locating and testing newly discovered sets of MZA would be mentioned in the diary, if this actually occurred. Their complete absence in the diaries would seem to be damning evidence. However, when the diaries are closely examined, as they were by Joynson (1989) and Fletcher (1991) (whose book also reproduces all the entries in Burt's diary for one full month), this negative evidence of not having collected any new sets of twins at least after 1953 suddenly becomes unimpressive. The reason is that Burt's diaries seem to record *nothing but* utter trivia; for example, there is no mention at all of the death of Burt's personal secretary of many years or of Burt's attending her funeral, which other records show he did. The diaries read more like a simple date book, with the briefest possible notations. What's more, some 55% of all the dates during the whole period covered by the diaries show no entries at all, and there are periods of several consecutive months without a single entry. So the mere absence of mentioning MZAs (or other kinship data) in the diaries, and the lack of any metnion of his former assistants, Howard and Conway, becomes a very unconvincing item of evidence for the charge that Burt faked his data. Yet it was Hearnshaw's rather misleading report of the nature of these diaries that had finally convinced almost everyone that Burt had committee fraud.

The nearest thing to a "smoking pistol" in Burt's diaries is the single entry, "calculating data on twins for Jencks," (Hearnshaw, 1979, p. 247). This item does give the reader pause. In 1968 Christopher Jencks, a Harvard sociologist, had requested from Burt a listing of the IQs and socioeconomic ratings of each of the 53 MZA twin pairs on which the correlations were based in Burt's important 1966 article. The crucial question here is Does "calculating data" mean deliberately *concocting data* to fit the already published correlations and other statistics? Or could it mean something else, perhaps just assembling data from various other tables or test sheets, or matching up the socioeconomic information on the subjects from separate data files? No one really knows. The indisputable evidence from Burt's correspondence that he told "white lies" to Jencks (and other correspondents) about the reasons for his delayed replies to their inquiries, such as being out of town, can hardly be construed as evidence that he fabricated the MZA data he sent to them.

Another source of suspicion, although perhaps not a smoking

pistol, is that Burt wrote to Professor Sandra Scarr, a noted behavior geneticist then at the University of Minnesota, in reply to her request for a copy of his data on 53 sets of MZA twins. In his letter, he also gave the IQs and other details on *three new sets* of MZA twins. (Scarr had sent me a copy of this letter, which I passed on to Hearnshaw.) I was especially puzzled by this, because about two months *after* Burt wrote that letter, I was personally discussing twin research with Burt and had even mentioned the possibilty of looking for more sets of MZAs in London. Yet he never mentioned having found the three new sets of twins he had described to Professor Scarr. It seems improbable to me to attribute Burt's silence on this point to a lapse of memory because, although he was then 88 years old, his memory was phenomenal for a great many other things, such as the technical details of one of my own studies that I had described in conversations with him 2 weeks previously. But again, this is inconclusive negative evidence.

THE CASE FOR THE DEFENSE

It is impossible in this brief account to do justice either to the great wealth of detail in Hearnshaw's biography or to the extensive and fine-grained investigation presented by Burt's defenders, Joynson (1989) and Fletcher (1991), hereafter referred to simply as J&F. Consequently, the case for the defense can only be characterized in the most general terms. But I first should confess that after reading (and even extolling [Jensen, 1983]) Hearnshaw's biography, the impressive case for Burt's defense presented by J&F was hardly imaginable. Until the shock and surprise of what is revealed by these investigations, I was fully resigned to accepting Hearnshaw's judgment of Burt's culpability (e.g., Jensen, 1981, pp. 124–127; 1983). Hearnshaw (1990) and the Clarkes (1990a, 1990b) have had a chance to respond to Joynson's (1989) analysis, and Joynson (1990) has answered. I found nothing in this rather sharp exchange that should rightfully put Joynson on the defensive, and he comes out looking even somewhat better, compared to Hearnshaw's attempt to refute him, than I might have expected.

The line of defense argued by J&F consists of two main tactics: (1) showing the previously unsuspected flimsiness, misrepresentation, and even in some cases factual nonexistence, of the supposedly damning evidence; and (2) closely examining the points that had aroused suspicions and providing alternative innocent explanations that seem at least as plausible as the "guilty" explanations promoted by Burt's accusers. The following paragraphs briefly consider the principal accusations and the counters put forth in J&F.

Point 1

Burt's assistants Howard and Conway could not be found, nor could their existence at any time be definitely established.

Counterpoint 1

Howard and Conway presumably worked for Burt only prior to World War II and, assuming they were still alive when sought in 1976, they would have been quite elderly. Burt's secretary testified that he had told her that Conway had emigrated, perhaps to Australia. Other persons that Burt mentioned in his articles and who at first were also suspected of being fictitious were later identified, and Fletcher (1991, Appendix 1) shows an example of the inability of the BPS to provide evidence of the existence of a former distinguished member whose obituary had recently appeared in the *Bulletin* of the BPS. However, it is important to note that Burt's articles were not explicit about exactly when Howard and Conway actually collected the twin data, and he was perhaps deceptive in leaving the impression that they were still giving IQ tests to twins even after 1955. My own hunch is that his personal vanity made him want to appear to be more actively engaged in ongoing research in his old age than he actually was, and so he obscured the "when and how" of his data collection, an implicit deception that later engendered doubts about the data's authenticity.

Point 2

Neither Burt's diaries nor correspondence provide evidence that Burt or any identifiable former assistants tested any new sets of MZ twins after Burt officially retired in 1950. Yet he added new twin data to his studies published in 1955 and again in 1966.

Counterpoint 2

Virtually all of Burt's data were collected before World War II. After the first blitzkrieg on London, University College had to be rapidly evacuated. All of Burt's data were hastily thrown into various boxes and stored in the basement, his department was moved to Wales for the duration; and in a later bombing raid, the College suffered a direct hit. One of Burt's long-time associates, Charlotte Banks, testified that the twin data were retrieved piecemeal after the war, in different boxes and at different times. Some of it had been misplaced and was turned up only much later (Joynson, 1989, p. 179). Alhtough Burt's articles implicitly made it appear that he was collecting new data, actually he only analyzed and reported for the first time old data that had been collected many years before. Burt's curious furtiveness in this regard undermined his posthumous reputation. But regardless of whether Point 2 or its Counterpoint is accepted, Burt's deception is inexcusable for a scientist. Many would say his reputation deserves the damaging consequences of such infidelity.

Point 3

Hearnshaw accused Burt of falsifying the history of factor analysis, belittling Charles Spearman's claims as the inventor of this technique, assigning major credit to Karl Pearson, the "father of mathematical statistics," and aggrandizing his own contribution to the development of factor analysis.

Counterpoint 3

Actually, Burt's account of the history of factor analysis is correct, and Hearnshaw's verdict on this score is simply mistaken (Blinkhorn, 1989). Pearson, in 1901, invented what today is known as principal axes or principal components analysis, although Pearson did not apply it to psychological data. But this technique was, and still is, widely used in psychological research, and it closely resembles virtually all other present-day methods of factor analysis. In contrast, Spearman's original method of factor analysis has been obsolete for more than 50 years and is seldom explicated in modern textbooks of factor analysis. Invented independently of Pearson's contribution a few years later, Spearman's formulas are no longer used, because they can extract only a single factor (a general factor, or g) from a correlation matrix and the method is correctly applicable only to a limited class of matrices (viz., hierarchical matrices with a rank of unity[3]). Burt's contribution occurred later, with the invention of a method of multiple factor analysis known as "simple summation." This method is similar to the "centroid" method later developed by Thurstone. In the days of mechanical calculators, both Burt's and Thurstone's methods had the advantage of being less laborious to compute than Pearson's principal axes. Hence, they were widely used for many years until the advent of electronic computers made mathematically more elegant and exact procedures practicable.

Point 4

In a feature article in *Science*, an American psychologist, Dorfman (1978), statistically demonstrated the fraudulent nature of data from one of Burt's articles on social mobility and IQ, which showed results consistent with the hypothesis that the average social class differences in IQ reflect genetic differences. Dorfman used Burt's bivariate (i.e., IQ × social class) frequency tables for parents and children to argue that the data in these tables fit the normal curve so closely as to be almost certainly faked. In other words, it was improbable that

---

[3]The clearest discussion of the limitations of Spearman's method of factor analysis that I have found in the literature is by Thurstone (1947, Ch.XII, especially pages 279–281). He states (p. 268) that the method is applicable only to a matrix of unit rank (i.e., a matrix with only a single-common-factor when communalities are in the diagonal) and also that, after solving for the first factor loadings by Spearman's single-factor formulas, attempts to extract additional factors in the same manner from the residuals will yield theoretically incorrect solutions; he presents a mathematical proof of this conclusion (p. 280). He notes that the application of the single-factor formulas to a correlation matrix can be justified only by regarding the result as a single-factor description of the correlation matrix. In that case the first-factor residuals are regarded merely as variable errors, which, if the matrix was not of unit rank, would be too large to be acceptable by Spearman's criterion of "vanishing tetrads." The method is obviously stymied in the face of a matrix of correlations that reflect multiple factors. In practice, Spearman always began his analysis by using his vanishing tetrads criterion for discarding any variables in the correlation matrix that broke its hierarchical pattern, or unit rank, before applying his formulas for calculating the variables' loadings on the single, or general, factor in the matrix.

random subject samples would show the high degree of regularity seen in Burt's tables.

Counterpoint 4

Apparently Dorfman's haste (as well as that of the *Science* referees who recommended publication of hs critique) to prove Burt a fraud precluded his reading Burt's article carefully. In it Burt explicitly indicated that he normalized the data and expressed them as relative frequencies to a base of 1000. Two professors of mathematical statistics, at Harvard and the University of Chicago, first independently then jointly, refuted Dorfman's effort. They pointed out that Burt's procedure of normalizing the frequencies, or fixing the marginal totals, was a statistically acceptable and not uncommon practice for this type of analysis (Rubin, 1979; Stigler, 1979). Jointly, they further stated that "using Dorfman's inappropriate statistical techniques to detect fraudulent data would be to condemn a major portion, if not all, of empirical science as fabrication" (Rubin & Stigler, 1979, p. 1206).

Point 5

In a claim they later repeated many times in print and on radio, Ann and Alan Clarke disclosed to Hearnshaw that Burt had published *articles* (solely under their names) based on their doctoral dissertations and that he distorted their views, in particular "implicitly attacking Eysenck" (Hearnshaw, 1979, p. 148).

Counterpoint 5

These alleged "articles" turn out to be nothing more than brief abstracts of the Clarkes' PhD dissertations. It was customary for professors to submit their students' dissertation abstracts for publication in the *British Journal of Educational Psychology*. Fletcher (1991, pp. 120–122) shows Alan Clarke's own typewritten abstract taken from his dissertation along with the published version in the *BJEP*. Burt had edited his student's abstract stylistically, as any good professor would do, and quite conspicuously improved it. There is no sign of any misrepresentation of the substantive content of the original abstract. Ann Clarke's (née Gravely's) dissertation did not have an abstract, so Burt wrote one for her, and it was published with her as the sole author. Joynson (1989, p. 246) checked the published abstract against the full dissertation and concluded that it is an accurate summary, with no sign of the alleged distortion. One may wonder if Hearnshaw bothered to check the Clarkes' misleading claim that Burt had written articles slanted against Eysenck under their own names, and if he did, why he did not question their guidance and advice (see note of acknowledgment in Hearnshaw, 1990, p. 61). The motivation of the Clarkes' prominent role in the Burt affair is still an enigma. They have yet to add any new evidence against Burt more substantial than this petty fizzle, which hardly seems a reasonable explanation for such gross vituperation. It is all the more puzzling since, whatever was the Clarkes' obscure motivation, unlike most of Burt's detractors, they are avowedly not antihereditarian and do not appear to be extremists on any of the related scientific issues. Yet, like a Wagnerian leitmotiv, Ann clarke's voice especially has resounded repetitiously as Burt's nemesis.

CONCLUSION

A moral of this curious story would seem to be this: If a scientist, for whatever reason, makes a good many personal enemies, works largely alone, is furtive, careless, or eccentric in the presentation style of his or her studies, and has become a prominent public figure; and, especially, if such a scientist's theories or findings involve ideologically or socially sensitive issues and happen to come out on the wrong side of popular prejudice to boot—then a store of excessive liability awaits a cabal of motivated opponents, avidly aided by the mass media, to bash that scientist's reputation completely.

This, I believe, is the essence of the Burt affair. Certainly, some of the accusations and suspicions leveled against Burt have been convincingly disproved by Joynson (1979) and Fletcher's (1991) effort's, though not all, and not completely, thus leaving room for doubt. Whether to give the benefit of the doubt to Burt or to his detractors is still another matter. Defending Burt convincingly is handicapped by his undisputed personal eccentricities and petty foibles, as well as by his failings as an empirical scientist. Because it is next to impossible to prove a negative, no one can confidently proclaim Burt's complete innocence of all charges. But the burden of proof rests squarely on those who have proclaimed Burt guilty of fraud. Their evidence has proven so flimsy that an impartial jury's careful examination of it would probably rule out the verdict of "fraud," not just as being "not proven," but even as being implausible.

It is hardly likely that anyone will utter the final word on the Burt affair, and I myself would not hope to do so. Although this extraordinary episode in the history of behavioral science has already consumed a great many gallons of ink, the future will very likely lavish many more. For better or worse, Cyril Burt's immortality in the annals of science is assured.

REFERENCES

Association of Educational Psychologists (1983). Sir Cyril Burt—The essential man. *Journal of the Association of Educational Psychologists, 6* (No. 1), 1–77.

Beloff, H. (1980). A balance sheet on Burt. *Bulletin of the British Psychological Society* (Supplement), *33*, i, 1–38.

Blinkhorn, S. (1989). Was Burt stitched up? (Review of *The Burt Affair* by R. B. Joynson). *Nature, 340*, 439–440.

Bouchard, T. J., Jr., Lykken, D. T., McGue, M., Segal, N. L., & Tellegen, A. (1990). Sources of human psychological differences: The Minnesota study of twins reared apart. *Science, 250*, 223–228.

Cattell, R. B. (1980). Review of "Cyril Burt, psychologist" by L. Hearnshaw. *Behavior Genetics, 10*, 317–325.

Clarke, A., & Clarke, A. (1990a). The Burt affair (Letters). *The Psychologist: Bulletin of the British Psychological Society, 2*, 74.

Clarke, A., & Clarke, A. (1990b). Review of Joynson (1989). *British Journal of Educational Psychology, 60*, 122–124.

Cronbach, L. J. (1979). Review of Hearnshaw (1979). *Science, 206*, 1392–1394.

Devlin, T. (1976). Theories of IQ pioneer 'completely discredited.' *Times*, October 25.

Dorfman, D. D. (1978). The Cyril Burt question: New findings. *Science, 201*, 1177–1186.

Evans, P. (1977). An interview with Jack Tizard. *APA Monitor, 8* (Nos. 9 & 10), 4–5.

Eysenck, H. J. (1939). Review of L. L. Thurstone's "Primary mental abilities." *British Journal of Educational Psychology, 9*, 270–276.

Eysenck, H. J. (1977). The case of Sir Cyril Burt. *Encounter, 47*, 79–91.

Eysenck, H. J. (1980a). Professor Sir Cyril Burt and the inheritance of intelligence: Evaluation of a controversy. *Zeitschrift für Differentielle und Diagnosticshe Psychologie, 3* 183–199.

Eysenck, H. J. (1980b). Psychology of the scientist: XLIV. Sir Cyril Burt: Prominence versus personality. *Psychological Reports, 46*, 893–894.

Eysenck, H. J. (1982). Burt's warped personality led inevitably to fraud. *The Listener*, (April 29), 2–3.

Eysenck, H. J. (1983). Sir Cyril Burt: polymath and psychopath. *Journal of the Association of Educational Psychologists, 6*, 57–63.

Eysenck, H. J. (1989). Sensitive intelligence issues. (Review of *The Burt Affair*, by R. B. Joynson). *The Spectator*, (December 2), 26–27.

Fletcher, R. (1987). The doubtful case of Cyril Burt. *Social Policy and Administration, 21*, 40–57.

Fletcher, R. (1991). *Science, ideology and the media: The Cyril Burt scandal.* New Brunswick, NJ: Transaction Books.

Gillie, O. (1976a). Crucial data was faked by eminent psychologist. London: *Sunday Times*, 24 October.

Gillie, O. (1976b). *Who do you think you are?* London: Hart Davis/MacGibbon.

Hearnshaw, L. S. (1979). *Cyril Burt, psychologist.* Ithaca, NY:Cornell University Press.

Hearnshaw, L.S. (1990). The Burt Affair—A rejoinder. *The Psychologist: Bulletin of the British Psychological Society, 2*, 61–64.

Hudson, L. (1972). *The cult of the fact.* London: Cape.

Jensen, A. R. (1972). Sir Cyril Burt: Obituary. *Psychometrika, 37*, 115–117.

Jensen, A. R. (1974). Kinship correlations reported by Sir Cyril Burt. *Behavior Genetics, 4*, 1–28.

Jensen, A. R. (1977). Did Sir Cyril Burt fake his research on the heritability of intelligence? *Phi Delta Kappan, 56*, 471, 492.

Jensen, A. R. (1978). Sir Cyril Burt in perspective. *American Psychologist, 33*, 499–503.

Jensen, A. R. (1981). *Straight talk about mental tests.* New York: Free Press.

Jensen, A. R. (1983). Sir Cyril Burt: A personal recollection. *Journal of the Association of Educational Psychologists, 6*, 13–20.

Joynson, R. B. (1989). *The Burt affair.* London: Routledge.

Joynson, R. B. (1990). The Burt affair—A reply. *The Psychologist: Bulletin of the British Psychological Society, 2*, 65–67.

Kamin, L. J. (1974). *The Science and Politics of IQ.* New York: Wiley (Penguin ed., 1977).

Newman, H. H., Freeman, F. N., & Holzinger, K. J. (1937). *Twins: A study of heredity and environment.* Chicago: University of Chicago Press.

Plomin, R. (1987). Genetics of intelligence. In S. Modgil & C. Modgil (Eds.), *Arthur Jensen: Consensus and controversy.* New York: Falmer Press.

Plomin, R. (1990). The inheritance of behavior. *Science, 248,* 183–188.

Rubin, D. B. (1979). Correspondence. *Science, 204,* 245–246.

Rubin, D. B., & Stigler, S. M. (1979). Correspondence. *Science, 205,* 1204–1206.

Stigler, S. M. (1979). Correspondence. *Science, 204,* 242–245.

Thurstone, L. L. (1947). *Multiple factor analysis.* Chicago: University of Chicago Press.

Vernon, P. E. (1972). *Cyril Lodowic Burt: A biographic memoir.* National Academy of Education.

Vernon, P. E. (1987). Burt, Cyril L. In R. J. Corsini (Ed.), *Concise Encyclopedia of Psychology* (p. 159). New York: Wiley.

Wade, N. (1976). IQ and heredity: Suspicion of fraud beclouds classic experiment. *Science, 194,* 916–919.

Personality Factors in Scientific Fraud and Misconduct

DAVID J. MILLER, PhD

INTRODUCTION

This chapter will explore what may be conceptualized as stable traits that may make certain researchers more vulnerable to committing scientific fraud or misconduct. Such inquiry is timely because recently there has been increased public (e.g., Broad, 1991; Broad & Wade, 1982) and professional (e.g., Verdict in sight, 1991; Kohn, 1988) interest in scientific misconduct and fraud. Chapter 9 of this book provides a comprehensive overview of academic pressures that

---

I would like to thank Drs. Samuel Popkin and Francis Dannenberg for their comments.

may, in subtle fashion, lead some researchers to commit fraud or misconduct. Chapters 4, 5, and 6 detail specific cases of admitted or alleged scientific fraud and misconduct.

The actual occurrence of fraud or misconduct is generally considered to be small, and until recently perpetrators were believed to be criminally responsible or to be suffering from some uncontrollable mental disturbance (Hilgartner, 1990). For example, Dr. Philip Handler, President of the National Academy of Sciences, has argued, "One can only judge the rare acts that have come to light as psychopathic behavior originating in minds that have made very bad judgments—ethics aside—minds which in at least this one regard may be considered deranged" (quoted in Woolf, 1981, p. 10). However, on further reflection, the scientific community has broadened the scope of responsibility for unethical conduct and acknowledged the potential for an institutional role. Specifically, the Institute of Medicine report on Responsible Conduct of Research (1989) pointed out:

> Investigations of cases of scientific fraud suggest that various factors in the research environment may contribute to the occurrence of scientific misconduct *even though they are not the direct causes of these occurrences* [italics added]. Examples, include pressures to "publish or perish," and emphasis on competition and secrecy in research performance, and inadequate interaction of young researchers with their peers and mentors. There is concern that not only ethics but also the quality of scientific research in general may suffer in this environment. (p. 1)

Despite the potential of institutional pressures, the individual researcher is still seen as ultimately responsible for his or her professional conduct. Whereas it is possible to explore why researchers may commit professionally unethical behavior, it is inappropriate to generalize about how they may conduct their lives outside the scientific realm. Hence, this chapter will limit the scope of its inquiry to those factors about questionable behavior that have been open to the public record.

"PERSONALITY" DEFINED

Braunwald (Chapter 4) states, "We must look to the behavioral sciences to help explain the deeper motivations for the commitment of research fraud, especially when it is gross and widespread.'' Although such examination may be of great utility, attempts at understanding the development and behavioral expression of personality differ widely. For example, from a psychoanalytic perspective, negative aspects of personality may be viewed as the expression of certain fixations in early childhood develpment, "primary process" activities, and defense mechanisms. Behavioral theorists, on the other hand, would avoid hypothesizing about inferred states or hypothetical constructs, would minimize the difference between various types of behaviors (e.g., adaptive vs. pathological), and would focus instead on schedules of reinforcement. Social learning theorists would emphasize the situational determinants of behavior and posit little evidence for the existence of enduring personality traits. Even though *personality* remains a controversial construct, a useful definition is provided by Maddi (1976), who views it as a ''stable set of characteristics and tendencies that determine those commonalities and differences in the psychological behavior (thoughts, feelings, and actions) of people that have continuity in time and that may not easily be understood as the sole result of the social and biological pressures of the moment'' (p. 9). Thus, an individual's personality may be thought of as that unique organization of consistent factors that generally characterize and influence his or her actions within the social and interpersonal environment.

ERROR, DEFENSE MECHANISMS, AND DECEPTION IN SCIENCE

Chapters 1 and 2 of this book present criteria for the conduct of moral or social behavior to which scientists are thought to subscribe, including Merton's criteria for universalism, communality, organized skepticism, and "disinterestedness." Merton (1957) also stated that instances of scientific misconduct were "deviant practices" and "should be seen in perspective." He implied that those instances were rare and that the scientific community supports and nurtures honesty and truth seeking:

Apart from the moral integrity of scientists themselves and this is, of course, the major basis for honesty in science, there is much in the social organization that provides a further compelling basis for honest work. . . . Scientific inquiry is in effect subject to rigorous policing, to a degree perhaps unparalleled in any other field in human activity. Personal honesty is supported by the public and testable character in science. (p. 651)

Of consequence, the *ideal* scientific "personality" is to be above reproach, exhibiting honest, open expression in the pursuit of truth (Knight, 1984). Nonetheless, the history of science is replete with mistakes. When examined retrospectively, numerous examples exist of scientists engaging in what might, at first glance, appear to be unethical behavior. However, researchers may publish erroneous data for a number of reasons (only some of which include the commission of scientific fraud). It is important to distinguish *error* from *fraud*, because if a scientist's impressions are eventually found to be incorrect, implications may arise that data collection, analysis, or reporting techniques were of a questionable nature. Scientific errors may be thought of as falling into three separate, although not mutually exclusive, categories: (1) conscious but erroneous conclusions based on mistaken, but honest, assumptions about the phenomenon being studied; (2) errors caused by unconscious or self-deceptive phenomena—the "human investigator" factor; (3) erroneous conclusions attributed to that which is traditionally thought of as fraud or misconduct in science (i.e., a conscious or deliberate attempt to mislead).

Honest but Erroneous Assumptions

For more than 2000 years, Western civilization held Aristotelian cosmology as *the* correct interpretation of the functioning of the universe. Aristotle placed the stars, planets, and sun all on a series of concentric spheres, which presumably circled the earth. Ptolemy then hypothesized that "epicycles" existed to account for anomalies in the Aristotelian system. Since the discoveries of Copernicus, scientists have viewed these beliefs as incorrect; however, they certainly do not condemn the pre-Copernicans for fraud. Researchers were simply conducting their observations and experiments based on what was, at the time, a common set of assumptions and the best data available. Although it is unfortunate that some scientists (such as Blondlot) hold onto a particular belief even after it has been disproved (see Chapter 1), professionals refrain from ascribing the label of fraud. Erroneous conclusions, in the absence of fraudulent behavior, may also occur if researchers are ignorant of accepted procedures for designing, collecting, analyzing, and reporting the results of a study. The research community should have in place proper academic training, mentorship, and safeguards (e.g., peer review, IRB and Human Subjects review, etc.) to protect against scientific inquiry by investigators who are unfamiliar with currently accepted standards. Although it is not fraud, plagiarism is often thought of as a form of scientific misconduct. It is important to recognize, however, that what we now accept as proper scientific etiquette may not have been the case in other social/historical contexts. For example, the extent to which background references were routinely acknowledged in ancient Greece, Rome, or Egypt is unclear.

Finally, a scientist can be duped. Broad and Wade (1982) report the unfortunate case of an 18th-century German physician Johann Beringer. Briefly, Beringer had developed a keen interest in archeology, which evidently had become common knowledge. In 1725, some local youths brought him a collection of stones and tablets that documented in Latin, Hebrew, and Arabic "the ineffable name of Jehovah." After Beringer published a book on the topic in 1726, he began to suspect foul play when one of the names etched on the stone appeared to be his own. An official inquiry revealed that two persons, a professor of geography and a librarian at the University of Wurzberg, had wanted to humiliate Beringer because "he was so arrogant." After the episode had been settled, scholars thought that Beringer might have been gullible and stubborn, but he was never accused of misrepresenting data that he believed to be true.

Thus, the reporting of erroneous data based on false assumptions about the phenomenon under investigation is not uncommon in the history of science. Scientists do not, nor should they, condemn individuals who openly follow the standards of currently accepted scientific practice—even if, upon reflection, they are wrong.

The Human Investigator Factor

When discussing alleged instances of scientific fraud and misconduct, it is necessary to ask two preliminary questions: Is there conscious awareness that some ethically questionable endeavor is being undertaken, and is there a deliberate attempt to misrepresent data or conclusions? In her philosophical treatise on deception and lying, Bok (1978) defines a lie as "any intentionally deceptive message which is stated . . . where the liar knows that what he is communicating is not what he believes, and where he has not deluded himself into believing his own deceits" (p. 16). She states that all deceptive messages, whether or not they are actually "lies," can also be more or less affected by self-deceit. In this realm, those "grey areas" between conscious intent and less than conscious behavior, lie the most complex (and sometimes perplexing) cases of misconduct and fraud. The following sections will briefly explore some potential explanations for why researchers may, without conscious awareness, commit fraud.

Reinforcement Theory.   Learning theory accounts for the possibility of less than conscious reinforcement of unethical behavior (e.g., Skinner, 1953). Blakely, Poling, and Cross (1986) state:

> Ethical training, in the form of punishment of deceptive behavior, is a substantial component of most scientists' operant history. Stimuli (including behaviors) correlated with the punished behavior come to function as aversive stimuli in that their termination or avoidance is reinforcing. One class of behavior most likely so correlated, and thus aversive, is self-observation of the fraudulent behavior. The aversive consequences of realizing that one is engaging in previously punished (i.e., deceptive) behavior can be terminated by turning one's self-observation elsewhere, which is thereby automatically reinforced. (p. 320)

Accordingly, when otherwise honest researchers engage in misconduct, self-observation of the unethical behavior becomes an aversive experience. By focusing on other actions, the researcher can avoid reflecting on his or her unethical conduct.

Actor/Observer Phenomenon.   Research in social psychology documents existence of what has been termed the "actor/observer" phenomenon. Specifically, individuals engaging in behaviors (i.e., "actor") make attributions about their behavior that focus on the external stimulus inherent in a particular situation. Those more tangentially involved in a particular situation (i.e., "observer") attribute particular behavior to more stable personality dispositions of the actor (Jones

& Nisbett, 1976). It also appears that salient features for the actor and observer are often quite different, and an actor may limit the scope of his or her data input. Hence, it would be possible for an individual to focus on external, institutional pressures (e.g., the awarding of a competitive grant, need to publish for tenure) for engaging in questionable scientific practices.

Psychodynamic/Developmental Influences. Braunwald, in this book and elsewhere (Braunwald, 1987) has outlined the case of Dr. John Darsee, who was a physician and fellow at the Cardiac Research Laboratory at Harvard Medical School. In Chapter 4, Braunwald, director of that laboratory, maintains that fraud represents "a form of unconscious self-destructive behavior, with aggressive components directed also toward colleagues, supervisors, institution, and society, all of whom are profoundly affected." Braunwald's conceptualization may have begun when allegations of misconduct against Darsee were brought to his attention. Briefly, Darsee published abstracts and papers subsequently judged by coauthors, collaborators, and the faculty committees at Emory and Harvard Universities, to represent, at least in part, unverifiable data and conclusions (Knox, 1983; Relman, 1983). When attempting to explain his behavior to the National Institute of Health, Darsee wrote a letter to the Deputy Director, who found it so "highly personal" in its references to the death of his father and his admiration for Braunwald that he has acceded to Darsee's request not to release it (Culliton, 1983).

Several factors in the case specifically deserve comment: (1) While at Emory, Darsee had apparently engaged in fraudulent behavior, prior to his relationship with Braunwald; (2) Darsee admittedly placed an unusually high value on his relationship with Braunwald; (3) Darsee evidently engaged in fraudulent behavior where he could be observed and discovered by others. There are at least two highly speculative, yet possible explanations. First, as Braunwald suggested, the death of Darsee's father in combination with subconscious awareness of his own ethical misconduct may have propelled Darsee into an angry, self-destructive pattern, which allowed observation of his behavior by others. Alternatively, after the death of his father, Darsee may have narcissistically overidentified with an overidealized father figure (i.e., Braunwald). Knowing the stature and reputation of his mentor, Darsee may have never entertained the possibility that his own investigations might be questioned. Therefore, he proceeded as though he were invulnerable to suspicion.

Modeling.   Social learning theory has consistently documented that individuals imitate valued models. When models demonstrate less than adequate research standards, students have limited opportunity to learn appropriate, ethical behavior. For example, when Dr. Elias Alsabti's mentor received substantial monetary support from the Iraqi government, he named two recently discovered anticancer drugs after his political benefactors. Unfortunately, when the (President Ahmed) Al-Bakr and (Vice-President Saddam) Hussein medications proved ineffective, he was not allowed to leave the country. Likewise, when Alsabti received monies from the same organization, he (reportedly) named a laboratory after the "Al-Baath" political party and a cancer detection method after President Al-Bakr. As with his mentor's discoveries, the effectiveness of the cancer-screening method has been challenged and even the existence of the laboratory has been called into question (for details see Chapter 5). Additionally, senior scientists working in governmental institutions may give priority to a political agenda rather than an empirically derived conclusion. Recently, the U.S. Department of Agriculture apparently "rephrased" the summary section of a major epidemiological study of the WIC (Women, Infant, and Children) program, resulting in the General Accounting Office maintaining that they "have not seen as blatant an example [of tampering] as this in twenty years" (Marshall, 1990). For young scientists within the Department of Agriculture, observation of this occurrence sets a dangerous precedent.

Cognitive Dissonance.   In 1957, Festinger proposed the basic theoretical assumptions of "cognitive dissonance" theory. The proposition is quite simple and basically states that an uncomfortable state of "dissonance" occurs when there is psychological inconsistency between cognitions. Festinger believed that when such dissonance occurs, a drive state is activated that attempts to return the organism to a baseline level of arousal. By resolving the inconsistent cognitions, the individual thereby returns to a state of decreased tension. Revisions of the initial theory (Aronson, 1969) state that dissonance is aroused when a person's core "self-concept" is threatened. When a person sees ego-inflation, monetary gain, power, or prestige the criterion for success, engaging in fraudulent behavior will cause minimal dissonance arousal. However, when a person's values are consistent with the scientific character (i.e., truth seeking as the ultimate goal) engaging in questionable behavior will arouse a great deal of dissonance. Hence, an individual may proceed to reduce the dissonance through a type of cognitive reframing or rationalization (e.g., "What will it hurt? . . . those would have been the results anyway").

Fraud, Misconduct, and Deception

Bok (1978) outlines various types of conscious deception, including "clear" lies with the intent to mislead, and "marginal" lies, where though not stated, the person's intent is to evade the truth or exaggerate his or her position. Often individuals offer the following explanations for avoiding personal responsibility when they have been accused or found guilty of misconduct or fraud.

"A Lie Is Not a Lie" but an Exaggeration or "White Lie." Examples of marginal lies through the alteration of ideas, data, or conclusions occur when a scientist "massages" (transforms the data to make that which is inconclusive appear clear), "extrapolates" (uses too few data points or misuses degree of variability of data), "smooths" (discards data that may be interpreted as statistical outlier), "slants" (emphasizes certain trends while discarding alternative interpretations), "fudges" (creates data points to complete data cells), or "manufactures" (creates a set of observations *de novo* without experimentation or observation).

In such cases, perpetrators often try to explain their behavior, for example, "I didn't make up anything . . . I simply took the mean ratings of the other data in the cells so I could perform the appropriate statistical tests." It appears that one of the great astronomers of all time, Johannes Kepler, resorted to this tactic when "instead of throwing it [anomalous data] out, he went back and tidied it up, made of it something quite different, covering up but not quite effacing the marks of his earlier struggle" (Donahue, 1988, p. 234). It would seem then that Kepler presented, as data, deductions from theory rather than observations, and he did so because of his concern that the entire Copernican system would be challenged. An additional factor may have been the general dissatisfaction with the prior treatment of his mentor, Tycho Brahe, for the reporting of "untidy" data. As we now know, it is fortunate that the theory that supported his *New Astronomy* was eventually put to the empirical test and proven correct.

Deceit Is Acknowledged but Agent Maintains Innocence.   Although the deceit is acknowledged as a lie, the agent maintains innocence because he or she is not really responsible for the occurrence. For example, genetic "hardwiring" that would mandate sociopathic, immoral, or mentally disturbed behavior would also exonerate the perpetrator from personal responsibility for it. In the late 1960s and early 1970s William Summerlin was involved in research investigating the rejection of organ transplants. His research involved placing the donor organ in a tissue culture prior to transplantation, with the hope of avoiding the immune reaction that would cause the organ to be rejected. His endeavors were scholarly and gained him a position as chief of a laboratory working on transplantation immunology at the Sloan-Kettering Institute for Cancer Research in New York. Problems began to arise when replication of his findings was not forthcoming and a laboratory technician noticed that purported skin grafts of black mice onto white mice could be removed with an alcohol solution. When confronted with this fact, Summerlin admitted to the Director of the Institute that he had used a felt pen to darken some of the black skin grafts on the white mice (Committee on the Conduct, 1989).

After Summerlin was suspended from his responsibilities, a six-member committee examined the work he had been conducting with rabbits as well as mice and also discovered errors in the reporting of results with cornea transplantation in rabbits. The committee then showed these findings to Summerlin, who admitted that he did not know which transplant procedures were carried out with which rabbits. Dr. Summerlin explained that his behavior was the result of "mental exhaustion" secondary to extreme professional and personal stress (Hixson, 1976). The National Academy of Science (Committee on the Conduct, 1989) reports that the investigating committee stated: "The only possible conclusion is that Dr. Summerlin was responsible for initiating and perpetuating a profound and serious misrepresentation about the results of transplanting cultured human corneas to rabbits" and characterized some of his work as containing "grossly misleading assumptions" (p. 15). The committee evidently entertained a mental disorder as an explanation for the behavior and recommended that "Dr. Summerlin be offered a medical leave of absence, to alleviate his situation, which may have been exacerbated by pressure of the many obligations which he voluntarily undertook" (p. 15).

Additionally, perpetrators of fraud often cite academic pressures or subtle, private sector influences. For example, in 1986 a group at Harvard's Dana-Farber Cancer Institute retracted a paper that had reported discovery of a new molecule that appeared to amplify the T-cell activities necessary for immune responses. Co-author Dr. Claudio Milanese admitted to fabrication of the data. In a letter to the senior author he stated that at first "I thought it was true. Then the cells stopped producing. There was a lot of pressure in the lab and I didn't have the courage to tell them" (Culliton, 1986, p. 1069). An article by Knight (1984) cites Farber (1983), who investigated the case of Dr. Joseph L. Cort. Dr. Cort was a researcher at Mount Sinai School of Medicine who evidently faked drug research data. Cort maintained, "I was under a lot of pressure and things got a bit confused. I had to earn the money for research or die" (pp. 434–435).

Research also documents that social affiliation or the need for approval may play an important part in obtaining desired results. In 1966 Rosenthal documented, in both animal and human studies, that communication of the experimental hypothesis to undergraduate research assistants can result in data favorable to that hypothesis. Thus, being aware of the positive ways in which completion of a successful research endeavor affects those involved, students or laboratory assistants may attempt to please their mentor through collecting data that would be favorable to a publication.

Researcher Offers Moral Reason for Misconduct. The researcher offers a moral reason why he/she lied by maintaining that a greater good (through avoiding harm or producing benefits) is served by altering the data or conclusions. Researchers who are passionately wedded to a particular theory may maintain a belief that they "know what is happening . . . there is unfortunately, no procedure to uncover the phenomenon." An example of "moral" misconduct to serve a "greater cause" would include the premature disclosure through the media rather than the usual peer-reviewed route because of the potential good of such early disclosure.

Additionally, a successful scientific career may be defined differently by different persons. For an individual researcher who fully realizes that international recognition is rare, the demarcation of success may be limited to the ability to provide a stable livelihood in a socially esteemed profession. If so, obtaining and publishing positive results may be seen as a way to secure a degree of self-inflation as well as monetary income. Knight (1984) notes:

> Individual success is given top priority as a cultural value because it is identified with self-esteem and self-worth: it is to modern man what religious salvation was to the citizens of the Middle Ages. Success in our day is essentially a matter not of achieving material gain but of acquiring security, in that the success is accepted as proof of one's own power, as perceived by oneself and others. . . . (p. 437)

Altering data in minor ways for studies to be published in minor journals (never to be referenced) may be a "safe" way for an individual to attempt a guaranteed income, either through a tenured faculty position or favorable comparison with co-workers.

Persons may also engage in fraud but publicly offer no reason. Dr. Robert Sprague became suspicious when coinvestigator Dr. Stephen Bruening claimed to have conducted studies during 273 days of a possible 261 work-day year (Committee on Government Operations, 1990). At the time, Bruening was employed at the University of Pittsburgh's Department of Psychiatry and conducted pharmacotherapy research with behaviorally disordered retarded children. Following an initial investigation by the University of Pittsburgh and a subsequent inquiry by the National Institute of Mental Health, Dr. Bruening pleaded guilty in Federal Court to falsifying much of his research. The University of Pittsburgh reimbursed $163,000 to NIMH for grant monies previously received, and Bruening was ordered to repay $11,352 in salary, serve 250 hours of community service, spend 60 days in a halfway house, and cease participation in any psychological research for at least 5 years. When asked to speculate about Bruening's motivation, Sprague has stated that he presumed it was for "the usual human desires—power, prestige, money, fame. The same reason people embezzle from banks, cheat on defense contracts, or cheat Wall Street" (Bales, 1988, p. 12).

CONCLUSION

The personal and professional norms publicly subscribed to by scientists are not unlike those of other professions "trusted" by the community. Like all other human endeavors, scientific inquiry is vulnerable to the foibles of human nature, is prone to self-deception, and is influenced by very powerful social incentives (e.g., materialism, power, fame), which may encourage deceit (Bok, 1978). Individual perpetrators of fraud or misconduct often state that they lack power and freedom within an organization to cope with the consequences of failure, such as social pressures, individual feelings of competition, or pressure from administrators to "cut corners." Nonetheless, the Institute of Medicine's (1989) conclusions are appropriate when they imply that individual researchers, regardless of why they behave as they do, are responsible for their conduct. Personal responsibility must be accepted by a researcher who fabricates a number, fills a cell, alters a subject's characteristics, copies from another's manuscript, or overgeneralizes conclusions. Individuals have the power to influence the amount of duplicity in their lives and must rule out deceit where honest alternatives exist (see "Symposium," 1991).

REFERENCES

Aronson, E. (1969). The theory of cognitive dissonance: A current perspective. In L. Berkowitz (Ed.), *Advances in Experimental Social Psychology* (pp. 1–34). New York: Academic Press.

Bales, J. (1988, November). Breuning pleads guilty in scientific fraud case. *APA Monitor*, p. 12.

Blakely, E., Poling, A., & Cross, J. (1986). Fraud, fakery, and fudging: Behavior analysis and bad science. In A. Poling & R. W. Fuqua (Eds.), *Research methods in applied behavior analysis.* (pp. 313–330). New York: Plenum Press.

Bok, S. (1978). *Lying: Moral choice in public and private life*. New York: Random House.

Braunwald, E. (1987). On analyzing scientific fraud. *Nature, 325,* 215–216.

Broad, W. J. (1991, March 17). Cold-fusion claim is faulted on ethics as well as science. *The New York Times,* pp. 1, 30.

Broad, W. J., & Wade, N. (1982). *Betrayers of the truth*. New York: Touchstone.

Committee on the Conduct of Science, National Academy of Sciences. (1989). *On being a scientist*. Washington, DC: National Academy Press.

Committee on Government Operations. (1990). *Are scientific misconduct and conflicts of interest hazardous to our health?* Washington, DC: U.S. Government Printing Office.

Culliton, B. J. (1983). Coping with fraud: The Darsee case. *Science, 220*, 31–35.

Culliton, B. J. (1986). Harvard researchers retract data in immunology paper. *Science, 234*, 1069.

Donahue, W. H. (1988). Kepler's fabricated figures. *Journal for the history of astronomy, 19*, 217–237.

Festinger, L. (1957). *A theory of cognitive dissonance*. Stanford, CA: Stanford University Press.

Hilgartner, S. (1990). Research fraud, misconduct, and the IRB. *IRB: A review of human subjects research, 12*, 1–4.

Hixson, J. (1976). *The patchwork mouse*. Garden City, NY: Anchor/Doubleday.

Institute of Medicine. (1989). *The responsible conduct of research in the health sciences*. Washington, DC: National Academy Press.

Jones, E. E., & Nisbett, R. E. (1976). The actor and observer: Divergent perceptions of the cause of behavior. In J. W. Thibaut, J. T. Spence, & R. C. Carson (Eds.), *Contemporary topics in social psychology* (pp. 37–52). Morristown, NJ: General Learning Press.

Knight, J. A. (1984). Exploring the compromise of ethical principles in science. *Perspectives in Biology and Medicine, 27*, 432–442.

Knox, R. A. (1983). Deeper problems for Darsee: Emory probe. *Journal of the American Medical Association, 249*, 2867–2876.

Kohn, A. (1988). *False prophets: Fraud and error in science and medicine*. New York: Basil Blackwell.

Maddi, S. R. (1976). *Personality theories: A comparative analysis* (3rd ed.). Homewood, IL: Dorsey Press.

Marshall, E. (1990). USDA admits "mistake" in doctoring study. *Science, 247*, 522.

Merton, R. K. (1957). Priorities in scientific discovery: A chapter in the sociology of science. *American Sociological Review, 22*, 635–651.

Relman, A. S. (1983). Lessons from the Darsee affair [editorial]. *New England Journal of Medicine, 308*, 1415–1417.

Rosenthal, R. (1966). *Experimenter effects in behavioral research*. New York: Appelton-Century-Crofts.

Skinner, B. F. (1953). *Science and human behavior*. New York: The Free Press.

Symposium on moral responsibility. (1991). *Ethics, 101,* 236–321.

Verdict in sight in the "Baltimore case." (1991, March 8). *Science, 251,* 1168–1172.

Woolf, P. (1981). Fraud in science: How much, how serious? *Hastings Center Report, 11,* 9–14.

The Consequences of Fraud

ALAN POLING, PhD

NULLIUS IN VERBA

Let me begin in candor. I once worked in good faith with Stephen E. Breuning, a researcher who falsified data concerning the effects of psychotropic drugs in mentally retarded people, and my name has appeared on publications containing data that he fabricated. That experience has taught me, in a way that no impersonal review of cases ever could, that the overall consequences of fraud in science are far-reaching, heinous, and irreparable. The purpose of the present chapter is to consider these consequences. In so doing, I will refer to illustrative personal experiences; I will not, however, review the Breuning case.

A brief consideration of the key words in the phrase "fraud in science" will set the stage for a discussion of the consequences of fraud. The word *fraud* stems from the Latin *fraudis*, which means a "cheating, deceit, or error." This meaning has been retained, and the *American Heritage Dictionary* (1988) defined fraud as "1. A deception deliberately practiced in order to secure unfair or unlawful gain. 2. A piece of trickery; a swindle.'' As used herein, fraud in science comprises activities that involve intentional falsehood, including but not limited to the fabrication or misreporting of data and procedures.

The word, *science,* comes from the Latin *scientia,* meaning "knowledge." But, as Peter Medawar (1984) explained,

> . . . no one construes "science" merely as knowledge. It is thought of rather as knowledge hard won, in which we have much more confidence than we have in opinion, hearsay and belief. The word "science" itself is used as a general name for, on the one hand, the procedures of science—adventures of thought and stratagems of inquiry that go into the advancement of learning—and on the other hand, the substantive body of knowledge that is the outcome of this complex endeavor, though this latter is no mere pile of information: Science is organized knowledge, everyone agrees. . . . (p. 3)

Fraud compromises science in every regard. Fraudulent practices are antithetical to scientific stratagems of inquiry, which demand honest descriptions of procedures used to contact natural phenomena, and of the results of those contacts. And fabricated data are not hard won; they merit no confidence whatsoever and have no rightful place in a body of organized knowledge. Given the foregoing, it is not surprising that fraud in science has undesirable consequences for many people.

CONSEQUENCES FOR THE PERPETRATOR

One person obviously affected by fraud is its perpetrator. If a researcher engages in fraudulent practices that are not detected, the end result is personal gain. The nature and magnitude of the gain depend on the specific malfeasance, but it is easy to imagine how a scientist could advance professionally by, for example, fabricating or laundering data. With professional advancement come a variety of rewards, including money and status. It is a reasonable surmise that the promise or achievement of these rewards induces some scientists to cheat.

But if a person engages in fraudulent practices that are detected, the end result should be personal loss. At a formal level, fraud in science is not tolerated. Most organizations concerned with the behavior of scientists, including universities, professional socities, and granting agencies, establish codes for ethical conduct and set penalties for breaking these codes. Moreover, some fraudulent practices are criminal. Nonetheless, there is no clearly established mechanism for dealing with suspected fraud in science, no assurance that it will be vigorously investigated and, if proven, appropriately punished. The manner in which a particular case is handled appears to depend on the evidence for fraud, the nature of the alleged misdeed, the status of the offending individual, and, perhaps most importantly, the characteristics of the person who suspects fraud. The Breuning case is revealing in this regard. By dogged persistence, Dr. Robert Sprague and a few associates forced an investigation that determined and made public the nature of Breuning's fraudulent practices and eventually resulted in criminal prosecution. Eventually, Breuning pleaded guilty to two counts of filing a false report and was duly penalized (Wood, 1988). Here, the consequences of fraud for the perpetrator were indeed serious. Beyond the formal penalties, Breuning's career as a behavioral scientist is effectively finished. Yet I wonder what the outcome would have been in the absence of a Robert Sprague.

CONSEQUENCES FOR COLLABORATORS

On first glance, it might appear impossible for a perpetrator of fraud to have collaborators, but they often do. In fact, of the manuscripts authored by Breuning that were reviewed for evidence of scientific misconduct by the Panel of Senior Scientists established by the Public Health Service, only two listed him as the sole author (Panel to Investigate, 1987). Of the remainder, 6 listed 1 coauthor, 8 listed 2 coauthors, 6 listed 3 coauthors, 1 listed 4 coauthors, and 1 listed 7. (Not all of these works contained data provided by Breuning, or gave evidence of misconduct.) The role of each coauthor is unknown, but it may be of interest to review my role in the empirical articles that I published with Breuning (Breuning, Ferguson, Davidson, & Poling, 1983; Davis, Poling, Wysocki, & Breuning, 1981; Poling & Breuning, 1983).

The Davis et al. (1981) article stemmed from an MA thesis conducted under my direction by Vicky Davis, who eventually married Breuning. The three of us designed the study, and we met on a regular basis to discuss it as it was allegedly being conducted. At the end of that time, I edited the thesis and helped to prepare the journal submission. I did not observe experimental sessions, but I did visit the study site (Coldwater Regional Center) and conduct trial sessions with the apparatus used to arrange the matching-to-sample procedure employed in the study.

With respect to the Poling and Breuning (1983) article, I played a role in experimental design and data analysis, and I wrote the manuscript. Breuning collected the data, which I saw only in summary form (i.e., as graphs). Some of the data were supposedly collected at Western Psychiatric Institute in Pittsburgh, with the remainder coming from Coldwater Regional Center. I did not visit either site while the study was ongoing. My role in the Breuning et al. (1983) study was minor. I assisted in designing the study, analyzing the data, and writing the report.

It is impossible to estimate accurately the time that I spent in working on the three articles, but it was considerable. Of course, early on the work was amply rewarded. Before Breuning's cheating was discovered, I received credit for being involved in what appeared to be exemplary research. After that, and rightly, the worm turned. In retrospect, every hour that I spent collaborating with Breuning, whether on empirical or review articles (Breuning & Poling, 1982; Breuning, Davis, & Poling, 1982), was worse than time wasted. Our interactions have tarnished my reputation and caused me pain. Much the same must hold for his other coauthors, and for the collaborators of other known charletans.

Despite being duped by Breuning, I continue to work with people that I cannot observe directly. Trust is implicit in such arrangements, but I do take care to require that collaborators provide me with full details concerning the conduct and results of studies. With Breuning, I asked for and received only global descriptions. Those descriptions were inevitably reassuring, but it is clear in retrospect that failing to ask for precise details concerning the conduct and results of studies was a naive and serious mistake. Although requiring such details does not obviate the possibility that they might be faked—a person could, for example, fabricate raw data—it does render a cheater's task more difficult, and it increases the odds of detecting irregularities in the conduct or results of an investigation. For these and other good reasons (Freedman, 1986), everyone who is involved in a study should be fully aware of, and satisfied with, all aspects of its conduct and reporting.

Even if the work is sound, it may be dismissed, if a known fraud contributed to it in any way. A recent article by Garfield and Welljams-Dorof (1990), entitled "The Impact of Fraudulent Research on the Scientific Literature: The Stephen E. Breuning Case," demonstrates this point. In that article, Garfield and Welljams-Dorof indicate (Table 1) how often 20 publications that Breuning coauthored were cited from 1981 to 1988 in the *Science Citation Index* and *Social Sciences Citation Index*. The implication, evident throughout the article, is that each of these articles is fraudulent. In fact, they are not. Consider, for example, an article by Wysocki, Fuqua, Davis, and Breuning (1981). The study on which that article was based was evaluated by the Panel to Investigate (1987). They concluded that:

> The article was based on the primary author's (Wysocki) doctoral dissertation. The data are presented in a straightforward manner. The Panel confirmed through its site visit to Coldwater and through interviews that this work was carried out as reported. (p. 23)

It is grossly unfair to consider this article, or others that are legitimate, as fraudulent simply because Breuning is a coauthor. Those concerned with fraud in science and its impact have an obligation to consider carefully whether the material that they consider is in fact fraudulent. Painting with a broad brush, in the style of Garfield and Welljams-Dorof, harms innocent collaborators and is unconscionable.

CONSEQUENCES FOR OTHER COLLEAGUES

To be harmed by fraud, it is not necessary for a professional to collaborate with a scoundrel. By cheating, an individual gains unfair competitive advantage over others working in the same research area. Grant money and journal space are limited, and the unethical researcher can control a disproportional amount of each by producing with ease what appear to be high-quality studies. Case in point: From

1979 to 1983, Breuning contributed 34% (24 of 70) of all publications in the area of psychopharmacology of mentally retarded people (Sprague, 1987).

Fraud in science may also do damage by opening false leads that are pursued by other scientists. If a researcher publishes interesting but falsified data, other investigators may attempt to replicate or, more probably, to extend those findings. These follow-up studies utilize time, effort, and other resources that could be put to better use. For example, consider parapsychology, a discipline in which fraud historically has been relatively common. It is so common, in fact, that Gordon (1987) pessimistically concluded, "Extrasensory perception, the so-called ability to perceive or communicate without using normal senses, would be better named extrasensory *deception*. The history of parapsychology, of psychic phenomena, has been studded with fraud and experimental error" (p. 13). Given this, it should come as no surprise that parapsychologists have wasted countless hours in the literal and figurative pursuit of ghosts (see, e.g., Kurtz, 1985).

An important digression: Although replication often is touted as a means of detecting fraud (e.g., Broad & Wade, 1982), it is not. The reasons for this are three. First, a researcher can present data that, although fabricated, portray a relationship that legitimate researchers can reproduce. Second, direct (i.e., exact) replication is relatively rare in science, unless the original findings are either of remarkable clinical or theoretical significance, or are highly anomalous in light of current theories. And, if a replication is not exact, it is difficult to determine what is responsible for a failure to replicate. As Barber (1976) noted:

> If an investigator in the behavioral sciences is unable to cross-validate an earlier study, the author of the earlier study will very likely argue that there were some important differences in the procedure which led to the failure to replicate. (p. 45)

In most cases, the author of the original study will not need to make such an argument, for the author of its sequel is likely to point out procedural variations that may account for the disparate results. Unless there is reason to believe otherwise, scientists must assume that their peers are honest; cheating characteristically is the last variable suspected to be responsible for unreplicable findings.

Fraud in science also extracts considerable opportunity cost from colleagues who review grant proposals and journal articles submitted by scoundrels, and from those who write reviews based on fabricated data. Consider, for example, a chapter reviewing pharmacological interventions with mentally retarded people that Michael Aman and Nirbhay Singh published in 1983. At the time of its appearance, the chapter was an excellent overview. Given the apparent methodological sophistication of Breuning's research, and the orderliness of his data, Aman and Singh rightly based some of their conclusions on his work. For example, they wrote the following:

> One way of increasing an individual's IQ score is by providing rein-forcement contingent on the correct performance on each test item (Clingman & Fowler, 1976). Recent studies have shown, however, that no such increases are to be found when the subject is on some form of antipsychotic medication (Breuning & Davidson, 1981; Breuning et al., in press [this is the Breuning et al. article published in 1983]) and that such an effect can be noticed even at very low doses (Breuning, in press [this article appeared in 1982]). Breuning et al. have suggested that medication impairs the subject's responding to external reinforcement. That is, antipsychotic drugs are said to interfere actively with the conditioning process and consequently reinforcement is believed to have a negligible impact on the test performance of these subjects. (p. 322)

The foregoing is an accurate assessment of the results of what appeared to be sound studies. But we now know that the data reported by Breuning were fabricated, hence the time Aman and Singh spent in reading, analyzing, and writing about Breuning's work was wasted. The same is true of anyone else who was concerned with Breuning's research, which includes almost everyone working in the area of drugs and mental retardation in the early 1980s.

Perhaps more importantly, the recognition that Breuning's work cannot be trusted has seriously eroded the data base concerning psy-chotropic drug effects in mentally retarded people. We now know less about how psychotropic medications affect this population than we appeared to know when Breuning's data was accepted. This has implications for patients, as well as scientists.

CONSEQUENCES FOR CLINICAL PRACTICE

Depending on the research area, scientific data may have direct, indirect, or no clinical implications. If fabricated data have clinical implications, their existence may lead clinicians to take actions not in the best interest of their patients. Consider, for example, Breuning's work concerning the effects of neuroleptic drugs on reinforcement-induced IQ (intelligence quotient) increases in mentally retarded people, discussed previously. Because much behavior is maintained by positive reinforcement and systematic educational programs based on it are often used with mentally retarded people (e.g., Scibak, 1983), it is crucial to know if and when neuroleptic drugs reduce sensitivity to positive reinforcement. Breuning's data at least intimated that such medication may generally decrease the sensitivity of mentally retarded people to positive reinforcement (Aman & Singh, 1986), which would constitute a serious limitation of the drugs. As Aman, Teehan, White, Turbott, and Vaithianathan (1989) pointed out,

> The reinforcement studies by the Coldwater group (Breuning & Davidson, 1981; Breuning et al., 1980, 1983) have been widely cited and have had considerable impact on professional attitudes towards drugs in the field (Aman & Singh, 1986a; Holden, 1987). As others have not been able to replicate the Coldwater findings, however, and given the finding of "serious scientific misconduct" with respect to much of Breuning's research (Panel to Investigate, 1987), it would be best to dismiss his claims on this important issue unless other workers are able independently to substantiate them. (p. 459)

The same is true concerning all other claims based on his alleged findings. Fortunately, it appears that the *general* conclusions supported by his data are reasonable with respect to clinical practice. In the reviews that I wrote with Breuning, which heavily emphasized his data, we stressed the following general points:

1. Neuroleptic (antipsychotic) drugs are potentially harmful and historically have been overprescribed for mentally retarded people.

2. Drug classes other than neuroleptics may be useful with some mentally retarded people. Drugs from these classes deserve further study, especially outside institutions.

3. Some mentally retarded people respond favorably to psychotropic drugs, others respond unfavorably. It is impossible to predict the response of an individual client prior to treatment; therefore, individualized and data-based evaluations are a necessary part of treatment.

We made several other points, but to me those three were primary. They are valid and clinically significant points that can be defended on the basis of data other than Breuning's (Aman & Singh, 1988; Gadow & Poling, 1988). But his remarkably orderly data, supposedly the result of methodologically sophisticated experiments, provided unequivocal support for those points. In the absence of those data, conclusions are necessarily weaker. For instance, it is abundantly clear that neuroleptic drugs can produce a range of adverse reactions (e.g., drowsiness and motor impairment) in mentally retarded people (Gadow & Poling, 1988), hence it is fair to state that the medications are potentially harmful. It is not, however, fair to claim that neuroleptics are harmful in reducing people's sensitivity to reinforcement, for this finding was supported primarily by data collected by Breuning.

Consider another example. Poling and Breuning (1983) supposedly examined the effects of methylphenidate on fixed-ratio lever-pressing by 12 mentally retarded children. Teachers' evaluations of behavior were also quantified via the abbreviated Conners' Teacher Rating Scale, which was used as a measure of clinical response. Reported results, now known to be fabricated (Panel to Investigate, 1987), indicated:

For five children, methylphenidate at oral doses of 0.3, 0.7, and 1.0 mg/kg produced generally dose-dependent decreases in response rates, whereas for the other seven children the two lower doses increased response rates while the highest dose decreased responding. (Poling & Breuning, 1983, p. 541)

Each child whose rate of fixed-ratio responding was increased by methylphenidate also demonstrated a therapeutic response to the drug. These data suggest that some mentally retarded children, perhaps those appropriately diagnosed as hyperactive, respond favorably to certain doses of methylphenidate. Some other studies support similar conclusions (see Gadow & Poling, 1988), but their results are less clear than those reported by Poling and Breuning (1983), and there is legitimate disagreement as to the appropriate role of methylphenidate in treating mentally retarded children and adolescents. It is unfortunate, to say the least, if clinical decisions in this area are based on the fabricated data that I reported with Breuning. *Even if the decisions are right, they are right for the wrong reasons.*

CONSEQUENCES FOR PUBLIC POLICY

Some scientific data have implications for public policy (e.g., concerning the kind of educational, medical, or social services that a government provides for its citizens) and, if the data are fraudulent, unnecessary or harmful policies may result. The case of the English psychologist, Cyril Burt, which is detailed in Chapter 6, provides an excellent example of educational policy being affected by fraudulent data. In brief, Burt (who died in 1971) steadfastly argued that intelligence was for the most part inherited. The validity of this hereditarian position was primarily supported by data from his own studies. Those data indicated that there was a strong positive correlation (about 0.77) in the IQs of identical twins reared apart (e.g., Burt, 1955, 1958, 1966). This correlation did not change across the course of several studies, in which the number of pairs of twins studied more than doubled to over 50. Such an outcome is so unlikely statistically as to be practically impossible. Leon Kamin (1974) noted this and other oddities in Burt's research, and strongly questioned the legitimacy of his data. It eventually became apparently to many workers in the field that those data were fraudulent, and they are generally discounted (Gould, 1981; Hearnshaw, 1979).

Burt's twin data had important implications for determining educational programs in England (Broad & Wade, 1982). His findings played a major role in establishing a system in which a child's performance on a test taken at 11 years of age determined subsequent school placement: Children who did well on the test received a higher-quality education than those who did poorly. Although Burt was not singularly responsible for this system, it is based on the notion that a child's capacity to be educated is essentially fixed and quantifiable, a notion strongly supported by his contention that the heritability of intelligence was over 0.75. That contention was supported by apparently fabricated data. Burt (1969) also used fabricated data to indicate that, after the system just described was replaced by a more egalitarian one, educational standards fell. The obvious implication was a need to return to the former, tiered system.

In the United States, Burt's data were used to argue that, because intelligence is primarily determined by heredity, programs of compensatory education are essentially useless (Jensen, 1969).[1] A related argument, to the effect that differences in social class are primarily a function of inherited differences in intelligence and are therefore difficult or impossible to change, also appeared (Herrnstein, 1971). These arguments have obvious implications for social and educational policy. In plain language, if intelligence is an essentially fixed, inherited quality that determines success in most areas of life, educational and social programs designed to improve the lot of the naturally stupid are doomed to fail. This contention is nonsense for many reasons quite apart from Burt's seemingly fabricated data (Gould, 1981), and there is sad irony in the fact that those data once added to its apparent credibility.

The relation between science and public policy is not one-way. Scientific findings determine public policy to an extent, but public policy also affects the activities of scientists. Well-publicized cases of fraud may suggest to citizens and elected representatives that much if not most of science is based on dishonesty, therefore it does not merit public support or acceptance. Such extreme skepticism would be an unfortunate consequence of fraud, for it is probably not warranted. As Peter Medawar (1984) noted,

> Enough examples of fraud in science have been uncovered in recent years to have given rise to scary talk about "tips of icebergs" and to the ludicrous supposition that science is more often fraudulent than not—ludicrous because it would border upon the miraculous if such an enormously successful enterprise as science were in reality founded upon fictions. (p. 32)

[1]Jensen indicated in a 1974 article that Burt's data were flawed and essentially useless, although he seems to have had second thoughts on the matter (see Chapter 6, this volume).

There is no doubt that science is enormously successful in providing a means of understanding natural phenomena. But the ubiquity of fraud in science is open to question. Known and egregious cases of fraud, such as those described elsewhere in this volume, are certainly rare. But those cases have garnered the attention of scientists (e.g., Maltzman, 1987), elected representatives (e.g., *Fraud in Biomedical Research,* 1981), and the news media (e.g., the Breuning case was considered on the CBS news program, *Sixty Minutes*). This attention may result in actions that reduce the future likelihood of fraud occurring, or increase the probability of detection and prosecution should fraud occur. If so, this is the one positive consequence of known cases of fraud in science.

CORRECTING THE HARM

In introducing this chapter, I stated that the consequences of fraud in science are irreparable. Surely that is true when individuals harmed by fraud are considered. It is perhaps hyperbole from a broader viewpoint. Science is not infallible, but it is self-correcting. If data are known to be fabricated, they will be rejected. Unfortunately, the knowing is a difficult process. And so is the rejection.

Consider the Poling and Breuning (1983) article, described previously. The study described therein was never conducted (Panel to Investigate, 1987). Given the publicity that the Breuning case has generated, it appears likely that researchers interested in the psychopharmacology of mentally retarded people know this today. But that was not true a few years ago. The Breuning case was investigated with glacial slowness. Well before the investigation was completed, I was convinced on the basis of interactions with Breuning and people familiar with him that the study was not conducted as described, if at all. Given this, on July 3, 1985, I wrote the following letter to the editor of the journal in which the article appeared:[2]

[2]On the same day, I sent a similar letter dealing with the Breuning et al. (1983) article to Daniel Freedman, the editor of the journal in which the article appeared. He and I corresponded at length, and eventually agreed that it would be appropriate to publish a retraction after the formal investigation was complete. My retraction (Poling, 1988), and retractions by Breuning's other coauthors, appeared in the *Archives of General Psychiatry,* accompanied by an introductory statement and an editorial by Dr. Freedman (1988).

In April of 1983, an article authored by myself and Stephen E. Breuning [reference provided] appeared in *Pharmacology Biochemistry and Behavior* (pp. 541–544).

Though I was the senior author of the article, the data reported therein were collected by Dr. Breuning. At the time the article was submitted for publication, I had absolute faith in their accuracy. Events within the past year have shaken that faith: At present, I cannot personally vouch that the study was conducted as reported in the article, nor that the data reported therein are accurate. I would like to inform readers of *Pharmacology Biochemistry and Behavior* to that effect but, given that Dr. Breuning does not share my concerns, am unsure how this could be done.

Any advice you might be able to offer concerning this sad and sensitive matter would be most appreciated.

The editor-in-chief of the journal, Matthew Wayner, replied:

Received your letter of July 3, 1985 concerning your manuscript [cited].

The circumstances which you describe are unusual. If there are inaccuracies or falsified data which invalidate or make the data which you reported unreliable, it is your responsibility to inform the scientific community. We would be willing to publish a "Statement of Author's Correction" in a forthcoming issue. If you can not resolve the difficulty with your co-author and publish such a statement jointly, then I would suggest that you contact the appropriate Ethics Committee of your respective professional societies for their evaluation and recommendation. If your co-author does not belong to a professional society, then I suggest that you contact appropriate administrative officials at the relevant institution and request that pressure be applied for compliance.

Please keep me advised of all further developments.

After corresponding, I spoke with Dr. Wayner by phone. The situation was clearly difficult. Although Breuning argued for the legitimacy of the data, I contended that they were at least flawed and in all likelihood fabricated. My contention was based primarily on the fact that Breuning had led me to believe that some of the data were collected at the University of Pittsburgh, with the remainder coming from Coldwater Regional Center. Subsequently, when under pressure, he related that most of the data were collected years earlier in the Chicago area, which was beyond belief.

But whether my misgivings justified a printed retraction was unclear to both Dr. Wayner and to me. The issue, of course, was one of standards of evidence. Beyond being highly unusual, a retraction by one of two authors without detailed explanation of the evidence supporting the need for retraction raised vexing legal issues. But a retraction with detailed explanation would be inappropriate given that the case was under formal investigation. In view of these considerations, it appeared best to withhold publication of a retraction until the investigation was completed. That occurred on April 20, 1987, when the final report of the Panel of Senior Scientists appeared. Shortly thereafter, Dr. Wayner moved to publish a retraction that I had prepared. Galley proofs of the following manuscript were mailed to me on June 25:

Editorial Note
The following retraction was first called to our attention on July 3, 1985 by Dr. Alan Poling. We decided that it would be best for everyone concerned to wait until a formal evaluation against Dr. Stephen E. Breuning had been completed. The report by the National Institute of Mental Health was made available on May 20 [sic], 1987.

Author's Retraction
Data reported in an article by Poling and Breuning [1983] appear not to have been collected as described, if at all [National Institute of Mental Health, 1987]. Therefore, it is my personal opinion that the article should not be cited, or used in any other way. I am sorry that the manuscript was ever prepared and sincerely apologize for any harm that may have resulted from its publication.

                                                                                Alan Poling

After I had returned the proofs, Dr. Wayner wrote to inform me that the retraction would not appear in *Pharmacology Biochemistry and Behavior*. To date, it has not appeared.

I relate this story not to criticize anyone—Dr. Wayner did everything in his power to help resolve the issue—but only to point out the difficulties intrinsic to dealing with fraud that is not admitted by its perpetrator. Neither collaborators nor journal staff have legitimate investigative status; they cannot resolve in any legally binding sense whether a given study is fradulent. And, unless fraud is duly proven, it cannot be formally reported without threat of reprisal. Even if fraud is clearly evident, as with the Poling and Breuning (1983) article, some publishers will, in apparent fear of lawsuits, fail to act. Others, however, will acknowledge the fraud. In one noteworthy example, the editors of *Research in Developmental Disabilities* (a journal in which two of Breuning's fabricated studies appeared), Johnny Matson and Stephen Schroeder (1988), published a retraction under their names. And recent reviews of pharmacological interventions in mental retardation characteristically indicate that Breuning's work is flawed and should be discounted (e.g., Gadow & Poling, 1988). Anyone with the slightest interest in mental retardation should be aware of Breuning's misdeeds.

But the Breuning case is a rare one in several regards, including the rigor of the investigation by the Panel of Senior Scientists, the strength of their conclusions, the criminal prosecution of Breuning, the penalties assigned him, and the media attention generated. It appears that many instances of alleged fraud in science are never investigated fully; others are investigated without satisfactory resolution (Broad & Wade, 1982; Kohn, 1986). In either case, data of questionable authenticity may retain an unmerited status as legitimate scientific information, and any harm resulting from their existence will go uncorrected. And that is certainly the case when fraud occurs but is not suspected.

A scientist who engages in fraudulent practices is not guilty of petty mischief that results in personal gain but harms no one. Fraud destroys the very fabric of science, and its consequences are as egregious as enduring. For these reasons, legitimate scientists must recognize fraud for the serious problem that it is. They must also be willing to confront it at the level of specific cases and general issues. Material presented elsewhere in this volume suggests that they are doing both with increasing regularity.

REFERENCES

Aman, M. G., & Singh, N. N. (1983). Pharmacological intervention. In Johnny L. Matson & James A. Mulick (Eds.), *Handbook of mental retardation* (pp. 317–338). New York: Pergamon Press.

Aman, M. G., & Singh, N. N. (1986). A critical appraisal of recent drug research in mental retardation: The Coldwater studies. *Journal of Mental Deficiency Research, 30,* 203–216.

Aman, M. G., & Singh, N. N. (1988). *Psychopharmacology of the Developmental Disabilities.* New York: Springer-Verlag.

Aman, M. G. Teehan, C. J., White, A. J., Turbott, S. H., & Vaithianathan, C. (1989). Haloperidol treatment with chronically medicated residents: Dose effects on clinical behavior and reinforcement contingencies, *American Journal on Mental Retardation, 93,* 452–460.

American Heritage Dictionary of the English Language. (1988). New York: Houghton Mifflin.

Broad, W. J., & Wade, N. (1982). *Betrayers of the truth.* New York: Simon & Schuster.

Breuning, S. E., & Davidson, N. A. (1981). Effects of psychotropic drugs on intelligence test performance of institutionalized mentally retarded adults. *American Journal of Mental Deficiency, 85,* 575–579.

Breuning, S. E., & Poling, A. (1982). Pharmacotherapy. In J. L. Matson & R. P. Barrett (Eds.), *Psychopathology in the mentally retarded* (pp. 195–251). New York: Grune and Stratton.

Breuning, S. E., Davis, V. J., & Poling, A. (1982). Pharmacotherapy with the mentally retarded: Implications for clinical psychologists. *Clinical Psychology Review, 2,* 79–114.

Breuning, S. E., Ferguson, D. G., Davidson, N. A., & Poling, A. (1983). Intellectual performance of mentally retarded drug responders and nonresponders. *Archives of General Psychiatry, 40,* 309–313.

Burt, C. L. (1955). The evidence of the concept of intelligence. *British Journal of Educational Psychology, 25,* 158–177.

Burt, C. L. (1958). The inheritance of mental ability. *American Psychologist, 13,* 1–15.

Burt, C. L. (1966). The genetic determination of differences in intelligence: A study of monozygotic twins reared together and apart. *British Journal of Psychology, 57,* 137–153.

Burt, C. L. (1969). Intelligence and heredity: Some common misconceptions. *Irish Journal of Education, 3,* 75–94.

Clingman, J., & Fowler, T. (1976). The effects of primary reward on the IQ performance of grade school children as a function of initial IQ level. *Journal of Applied Behavior Analysis, 9,* 19–23.

Davis, V. J., Poling, A., Wysocki, T., & Breuning, S. E. (1981). Effects of phenytoin withdrawal on matching to sample and workshop performance of mentally retarded persons. *The Journal of Nervous and Mental Disease, 150,* 718–725.

Fraud in Biomedical Research. (1981). *Hearings before the Subcommittee on Investigations and Oversight of the Committee on Science and Technology*, U.S. House of Representatives, 97th Cong., March 31–April 1, 1981. Washington, DC: U.S. Government Printing Office.

Freedman, D. X. (1988). Editorial: The meaning of full disclosure. *Archives of General Psychiatry, 45*, 689–691.

Gadow, K., & Poling, A. (1988). *Pharmacotherapy in mental retardation*. San Diego: College-Hill Press.

Garfield, E., & Welljams-Dorof, A. (1990). The impact of fraudulent research on the scientific literature: The Stephen E. Breuning case. *Journal of the American Medical Association, 263*, 1424–1426.

Gordon, H. (1987). *Extrasensory deception*. Buffalo, NY: Prometheus Books.

Gould, S. J. (1981). *The mismeasure of man*. New York: W. W. Norton.

Hearnshaw, L. S. (1979). *Cyril Burt, psychologist*. London: Hodder & Stoughton.

Herrnstein, R. (1971, September). I.Q. *The Atlantic*, 43–64.

Holden, C. (1987). NIMH finds a case of "serious misconduct." *Science, 235*, 1488–1489.

Jensen, A. R. (1969). How much can we boost IQ and scholastic achievement? *Harvard Educational Review, 39*, 1–123.

Jensen, A. R. (1974). Kinship correlations reported by Sir Cyril Burt. *Behavior Genetics, 4*, 1–28.

Kamin, L. J. (1974). *The science and politics of IQ*. Potomac, MD: Lawrence Erlbaum.

Kohn, A. (1986). *False prophets*. New York: Basil Blackwell.

Kurtz, P. (1985). *A skeptic's handbook of parapsychology*. Buffalo, NY: Prometheus Books.

Maltzman, I. (Chair). (1987, August). *Fraud in science: Is there self-correction?* Symposium conducted at the meeting of the American Psychological Association, New York.

Matson, J. L., & Schroeder, S. R. (1988). Editorial: A retraction. *Research in Developmental Disabilities, 9*, 1–2.

Medawar, P. B. (1984). *The limits of science*. New York: Harper & Row.

Panel to investigate allegations of scientific misconduct under Grants MH-32206 and MH-37449. (1987, April 20). *Final report: Investigation of alleged scientific misconduct on Grants MH-32206 and MH-37449*. Washington, DC: Public Health Service.

Poling, A. (1988). To the editor. *Archives of General Psychiatry, 45*, 686.

Poling, A., & Breuning, S. E. (1983). Effects of methylphenidate on the fixed-ratio performance of mentally retarded children. *Pharmacology Biochemistry and Behavior, 18*, 541–544.

Scibak, J. W. (1983). Behavioral treatment. In J. L. Matson & J. A. Mulick (Eds.), *Handbook of mental retardation* (pp. 339–350). New York: Pergamon Press.

Sprague, R. L. (1987, August). The myth of self-correcting science: Case history of reporting fraud. In I. Maltzman (Chair), *Fraud in science: Is there self-correction?* Symposium conducted at the meeting of the American Psychological Association, New York.

Wood, P. (1988, September 19). Guilty pleas in science fraud called victory for honest research. *Champaign-Urbana News Gazette*.

Wysocki, T., Fuqua, W., Davis, V. J., & Breuning, S. E. (1981). Effects of thioridazine (Mellaril) on titrating delayed matching-to-sample performance of mentally retarded adults. *American Journal of Mental Deficiency, 85,* 539–547.

System Considerations and Safeguards

CHAPTER 9

Academic Pressures

MARK H. THELEN, PhD
THOMAS M. Di LORENZO, PhD

INTRODUCTION

Decisions about whether research fraud occurs because of academic pressures can be made only after thoroughly understanding the immense variability in the definitions of fraud. Also, the wide variability in the estimates of the frequency of research fraud attributable to academic pressures appears to be related to the lack of an agreed-upon definition. This chapter will begin with a brief overview of the various definitions and prevalence estimates of fraud. Possible reasons for fraud related to academic pressures will be explored next. We will conclude with a section on directions for future research and suggestions for minimizing the incidence of fraud caused by academic pressures.

Definitions

The term *research fraud* has certain legalistic overtones that imply intent to deceive (DuBois, 1989), intentional misrepresentation (Engler, Covell, Friedman, Kitcher, & Peters, 1987), and carried with it the possibility of punitive consequences from outside the academic arena. Research fraud also implies gross mismanagement of the research endeavor (e.g., wanton and flagrant misuse of government funds). On the other hand, the types of activity that are considered to be incidents of research fraud have been viewed on a much wider continuum. Such variability seems to be captured in a related term that is used to describe fraudulent behaviors, as well as problems of misconduct and misrepresentation, *intellectual dishonesty in science* (Garfield, 1987, p. 3).

Garfield (1987) noted that various authors have drawn an obvious distinction between fraud and intellectual dishonesty or misrepresentation. Engler et al. (1987) made three distinctions. Inaccurate statements could be made:

(1) through justifiable mistakes—cases in which the scientist had no knowledge or basis for believing that the statements he or she was making were incorrect; (2) through careless errors—cases in which the scientist had no intent to deceive but the information that would have provided reason to doubt the accuracy of the statements made was available; and (3) through fraud—cases in which the statements made were known by the scientist to be false and in which the scientist intended to deceive others. Justifiable mistakes do not raise the issue of culpability. Careless errors and fraud involve a range of culpable actions, from negligence in the supervision of research or the execution of experiments to a clear intent to deceive. (pp. 1383–1384)

Although their definition appears to be somewhat concrete, making reliable classifications of specific behavior would be difficult. Blakely, Poling, and Cross (1986) noted two reasons that "make it difficult to discern whether a scientist's behavior involves premeditated intent to deceive" (p. 319). First, *intent* to deceive can only be inferred and not directly assessed. An individual who knowingly intends to commit fraud or misrepresentation will not only likely make attempts to cover up the incident(s) but also not admit to it later. Second, the individual may not be "aware of" or be able to report his or her fraudulent or unethical behavior. Although Blakely et al. (1986) provide an interesting "behavioral" description of how this may occur, they suggest that this type of behavior could be referred to as repression. For the above reasons, we will consider the larger gamut of behavior that may be subsumed under the terms fraud or intellectual dishonesty rather than behavior that represents a narrow definition of fraud (i.e., an intention to deceive).

Table 9.1 includes a variety of activities that have been labeled, or could be considered, as research fraud, intellectual dishonesty, misconduct, or misrepresentation. Huth (1986) noted that some abuses may not be "dramatically unethical" (p. 258). Indeed, "the scientific community might not ever agree on whether repetitive and duplicative publication are unethical. Wasteful publication might be seen as *jus-*

Table 9.1. Behavior That Could Be Considered as Fraud or Misconduct

Carelessness or bias in conducting or recording experiments	Relman (1989)
Fabrication of data	Merton (1957)
Fudging or suppression of data	Zuckerman (1977)
Commitments made in grant proposals	Harrobin (1989)
Incomplete authorship	Huth (1986)
Intentional efforts to communicate false or misleading findings	Bobys (1983)
Mismanagement of reporting scientific data	Szilagyi (1984)
Misrepresentation of data, research procedures, or data analysis	Mishkin (1988)
Multiple papers from one study	Huth (1986)
Neglect or violation of methodological concerns and procedural precautions	Zuckerman (1977)
Plagiarism	Merton (1957)
Publication of same material repeatedly	Huth (1986)
Selection and manipulation of results	Blakely et al. (1986)
Selective reporting of data	Mahoney (1976)
Slanderous charges of plagiarism	Merton (1957)
Stolen ideas	Steneck (1984)
Underacknowledgment of intellectual predecessors	Garfield (1980)
Unjustifiable authorship	Huth (1986)
Violation of federal, state, or institutional rules	Mishkin (1988)

tified by needs to compete for institutional and financial support to ensure academic survival" (Huth, 1986, p. 258, emphasis added). If "mild" cases of misrepresentation are viewed as acceptable or justifiable forms of behavior, it is easy to see how this viewpoint can lead to the assumption that fraud or more serious forms of misrepresentation may become necessary in view of academic pressures. The problem becomes more pronounced with the consideration that some individuals are unaware of the extent to which their actual behavior or practices deviate from accepted behavior or practices (DuBois, 1989; Mishkin, 1988). For example, Mishkin (1988) described an individual who was totally unaware of how his behavior deviated from generally accepted practice. She noted, "It seemed he believed (among other things) that it was permissible to draw graphs and charts *before* he had collected the data the figures were supposed to illustrate" (p. 1933). By considering the broadest definition of fraud, intellectual dishonesty, or potentially unethical behavior here, we can more easily postulate how academic pressures may play a role in their occurrence.

PREVALENCE

There is no known data base that would provide an estimate of the prevalence of fraud or misconduct in science. Broad and Wade (1982) indicate that there have only been 34 cases of fraud reported or strongly suspected from the second century through the early 1980s. Miers (1985) noted that the number of cases of misconduct in NIH-funded research is "almost insignificant" (p. 831) given the volume of funded research. However, Koshland (1987) noted that some newspaper reports suggest a much higher rate of fraud without mentioning that the amount of research conducted since the 1800s has grown exponentially. There are no data that would support an increased percentage of fraud today as opposed to 100 years ago. Miers (1985) offers relevant observations.

There is no question that the incidence of *reported* misconduct has increased dramatically. In the past three years, NIH has received an average of two reports per month of possible misconduct that appears to go beyond the traditional kinds of issues encountered in the fiscal and administrative management of grants, cooperative agreements, and contracts. About half of the reports have proven to be factual. Some of those reflected not fraudulent intent but some error in methodology or sloppy technique. Others appeared to be the result of the failure to develop and communicate appropriate policies and internal controls within academic and research institutions. The reports of misconduct cover a full range of behaviors. A few have involved possible egregious misuse of funds, but the majority are concerned with departures from accepted research practices, including fabrication, misrepresentation or selective reporting of results, inadequate attention to the rights of human subjects, and unacceptable treatment of laboratory animals. (p. 831)

As noted earlier, by broadening the definition of the types of behaviors that are being considered in this discussion, there may appear to be a greater prevalence of problematic behaviors in the academic endeavor. Petersdorf (1989) noted that fraud and misconduct have become major problems for both science and medicine:

It has been suggested that products of the system in which dishonesty is conducted are fair game to be seduced by the pressures of academia: the pressure to excel, the pressure to produce, the pressure to publish, the pressure to be promoted, and the pressure to cope with that academic albatross, the need to achieve tenure. Whether there is a connection between the early professional environment and research fraud is not clear. What is clear is that fraud is a major affliction of science and medicine. (p. 121)

For these reasons, it is clear that a thorough analysis should be conducted of the various academic pressures that may contribute to fraud or misconduct. The following sections explore the possible reasons for fraudulent research by academics. Specifically, what is the nature and extent of pressure in academia? What qualities within individuals might contribute to heightened stress or fraudulent behavior? And, finally, what external circumstances might increase academic pressure? Of course, factors within the individual can interact with external circumstances to increase academic pressure.

The research cited in this section often covers the entire spectrum of faculty who are employed in a university setting. Most of the studies and reports would have to be excluded if we reviewed only those that are of particular interest in this volume.

EXTENT OF STRESS AND PRESSURE IN ACADEMIA

Faculty responses to 23 items that assessed various aspects of morale revealed that a plurality of the respondents indicated that they experienced low morale (Hunter, Ventimiglia, & Crow, 1980). In a study of academic and applied psychologists, Boice and Myers (1987) reported that the academics had higher levels of health-related concerns, such as sadness and insomnia, than did the applied psychologists.

In contrast to these studies, two surveys indicated that academic faculty reported no more signs of stress than nonacademic control groups. Although 60% of the academic faculty showed physical signs (e.g., headaches) of stress, this was not significantly different from personnel in the student affairs office (Brown et al., 1986). Similarly, there was no significant difference on a measure of overall job stress between university faculty and a control group, matched on demographic variables (Horowitz, Blackburn, Edington, & Kloss, 1988). Finally, a study by Frazier, Morrow, & Thoreson (1990) reported no gender differences among faculty in level of performance, but females reported more stress than males.

Based on this research, it would appear unclear whether university faculty experience more stress than people in other work settings. However, it is possible to infer from the research that university faculty experience a high level of work stress. This might be particularly the case for female faculty.

PSYCHOPATHOLOGY AS A CAUSE OF STRESS

One approach to the problem of research fraud has been to suggest that the fraudulent person has some significant psychological and/or developmental problem. Based on this view, fraudulent behavior stems not so much from the circumstances that may generate high levels of stress, but instead from the psychological problems within the individual. The fraudulent behavior is a manifestation of those psychological difficulties.

One view of the problem of research fraud is to consider that a person who commits fraud is sick and to medicalize the problem.

Viewing the behavior as a sickness absolves the fraudulent person of responsibility for his or her actions (Fox, 1977). In contrast to Fox (1977), Woolf (1981) argued that research fraud is a form of psychopathic behavior. Presumably, researchers who commit fraud do so, not so much out of great pressure, but because it is an expedient way to reach their goals, and they perform this fraudulent behavior with little or no remorse. Knight (1984) questioned the explanation of fraud as psychopathic behavior and, instead, suggested that those who commit fraud have failed to reach the highest level of moral development.

Although not writing specifically about research fraud; Mahoney (1979) has had a different view of researchers and what makes them function as they do. Mahoney has argued that scientists are not always objective or open-minded in pursuing their research work. The tendency to be biased and to perceive selectively may be one reason why university faculty engage in fraudulent behavior.

PERSONALITY CHARACTERISTICS

In this section we will consider personality characteristics that may be associated with experiencing and reporting job stress. Several studies have been designed to examine performance and expectations among faculty as they might relate to stress. Brown et al. (1986) reported that 22% of the 191 faculty surveyed indicated high self-expectations. In a study of 1920 faculty, 53% indicated high self-expectations (Gmelch, Lovrich, & Wilke, 1984). Furthermore, there was a positive association between high self-expectations and high reported stress. Stumpf and Rabinowitz (1981) investigated the relationship between performance and job satisfaction at the various rank levels. The authors found that the high performers were the least satisfied, but this was true only among senior faculty. No such relationship was found among the junior faculty. These data were discussed by the authors in terms of the possible high expectations of some of the senior faculty resulting in both high performance and reduced satisfaction.

The research and theory on locus of control might suggest that "internals" would feel more in control of their work environment than "externals" and therefore more satisfaction with their job. This prediction was affirmed in a study by Shukla and Upadhyaya (1986).

Other researchers have studied a variety of personality attributes that might be related to job stress. Seiler and Pearson (1984) studied accounting educators. Their measure of stress contained several components (e.g., depression, physical exhaustion). Faculty who showed low self-confidence, inactivity, and low assertiveness reported higher levels of stress. Those who were goal-oriented reported higher levels of stress than their less goal-oriented counterparts. These data are somewhat consistent with the previously mentioned research concerning the positive association between self-expectations and reported stress. It might be inferred that goal-oriented people would have high self-expectations. On the other hand, those who are confident, active, and assertive may feel a greater sense of control in their environment and, therefore, feel less stressed. This observation would be consistent with the research on locus of control.

The final report to be reviewed in this section concerns another study with accounting educators (Seiler & Pearson, 1984). These authors reported that high-stress individuals, compared with low-stress individuals, showed more impatience, assertiveness, workaholism, and idealism. Again, there is some consistency in terms of behavior that is similar to Type A behavior and the indication of high self-expectations, which are all related to high stress.

The research reviewed here suggests that certain people may be more vulnerable to stress than other people, regardless of the circumstances in the work environment. We turn now to several aspects of the academic work environment that might contribute to stress among university faculty.

CIRCUMSTANCES CONDUCIVE TO STRESS

Even before taking an academic position, aspiring academics receive the message that they must be prolific in research. In a national survey of all PhD-granting experimental psychology programs, there was a significant increase (from 1982 to 1987) in the number of publications authored by the new PhDs that were employed (Follette & Klesges, 1988).

Medical students soon learn that fierce competition and pressure are a part of their schooling environment. Petersdorf (1986) has described the intense competition of the premed majors, which continues in medical school. This pressure may well be an important factor in the finding that 88% of the premed students surveyed had cheated and that many of these behaviors continued in medical school (Barrett, 1985). It is a reasonable possibility that this pattern of dishonesty may later be expressed in the form of fraudulent behavior while conducting research.

An increasing competitiveness to get an academic job has been documented by Bornstein (1980). Bornstein sampled a group of young psychologists (mean age, 33 yrs) and found that they published 2.2 times as much as their senior counterparts (mean age, 55 yrs) did early in their careers. Furthermore, the younger psychologists began publishing an average of 2.4 years before receiving a doctoral degree, compared with .7 years for the older sample.

Although the pressure to publish may take different forms, many researchers and writers have emphasized the strong relationship between publication rate and promotion and tenure (and to merit pay or salary). Several writers have argued that the pressure to publish research is strong and that it is probably a factor in research fraud (Bobys, 1983; Knight, 1984; Relman, 1989). Researchers have documented their untenured faculty report more stress than tenured faculty (Gmelch, Wilke, & Lovrich, 1986). It is likely that a significant reason for the stress among untenured faculty is the perceived pressure and uncertainty surrounding the granting of their tenure. The importance of research productivity to obtaining tenure is well known by anyone in or close to academia (Altman & Melcher, 1983; Gottfredson, 1978; Petersdorf, 1986; Scott, 1974).

The link between research productivity and salary is also common knowledge among those who are informed about the workings of academia. In a national survey of psychologists, Boice and Myers (1987) reported that 44% of the academic psychologists were concerned and stressed about salary, compared with 21% of the psychologists in private practice. In a factor analysis of a stress survey conducted with academic faculty, it was found that concern about perceiving adequate rewards was an important part of the stress (Gmelch et al., 1986). Consistent with the preceding finding, a survey of more than 1000 faculty revealed that 41% were stressed about the adequacy of their salary to meet their financial needs (Gmelch et al., 1984).

The importance of publishing becomes a source of pressure primarily to the extent that it is difficult to get research published. There is ample evidence that this is the case and, furthermore, that faculty are becoming increasingly prolific, thereby further increasing competition. A survey of researchers from 1965 to 1977 revealed that the average number of publications per year per faculty member increased for the physical scientists and life scientists and decreased for the social scientists (King, McDonald, & Roderer, 1981). Similar trends were revealed in a survey of all of the faculty in Minnesota from 1968 to 1980 (Willie & Stecklein, 1982). There were significant increases in the number of faculty who wrote chapters, books, and journal articles. Although many faculty are becoming more productive, it is becoming increasingly difficult to publish in the prestigious journals. Zuckerman and Merton (1971) reported that there is a decline in the ratio of the number of available pages in the prestigious journals to the number of persons in the social and behavioral sciences. The average rejection rate was 80%. A different survey of 540 journals in the social and behavioral sciences revealed a mean rejection rate of 76% (Mullins, 1977).

Assessments of the quality of research and the amount of productivity occur, not only at the peer review level by the journal editors and grant review committees, but also at the department and campus levels. It is likely that faculty ask how much research is required to get tenure, to get a good salary increase, and so on. However, departmental research requirements are often implicit and misunderstood by faculty (Woolf, 1986). Suggestions of bias have also been made concerning the peer review of research reports at the level of journal publication (e.g., Cicchetti & Conn, 1976; Cole, Cole, & Simon, 1981). The problem of evaluating research is further compounded by the diverse opinions as to whether a given outlet is refereed or not refereed: an important factor in the evaluation of quality (Miller & Servan, 1984).

Conducting and publishing research is not only important to tenure, promotion, and salary adjustments, it is also critical in obtaining and maintaining grant funding (Altman & Melcher, 1983; Begley, Hager, & Doherty, 1987; Rensberger, 1977). These observations are supported by a survey of a large number of faculty, the results of which revealed that 50% of the faculty indicated that financial support for research is a significant source of stress (Gmelch et al., 1984). Hence, the competition for grant funds and the research necessary to obtain grants are seen as a source of stress and the possible cause of research fraud (Petersdorf, 1986). Not only is the distribution of funds to individuals linked to research productivity, the distribution of funds to the departments on university campuses is increasingly linked to research productivity, and the amount and number of grants in the department (Wheeler, 1989).

Still another source of stress, which in turn might lead to fraud among university faculty, appears to be a perception of inadequate time to carry on all of the various duties, including research. Two studies have reported that time constraints and work overload are troublesome and conducive to stress (Brown et al., 1986; Gmelch et al., 1986).

We have documented the importance of research productivity to promotion, tenure, salary, and obtaining grants. In addition to conducting research, however, most faculty in college and university settings are expected to teach. If teaching is expected, but research is rewarded, faculty are likely to experience a conflict about how they should allocate their time between these two activities. It has been suggested that faculty are paid to teach but are evaluated on the basis of their scholarly works (Caplo & McGee, 1965). The faculty in one university believed that teaching was the most important activity; however, they realized that research productivity was given the most weight in personnel decisions (Hunter et al., 1980). This dilemma may be especially prominent among junior faculty who are striving for tenure and promotion. They may be most inclined to neglect their teaching duties in order to concentrate on research activities (Silver, 1983). The relative value of research over teaching, as evidenced by salary decisions, is documented in several reports. Each of these studies is based on data obtained from faculty or departmental records, and each shows a closer relationship between research productivity and salary than between teaching effectiveness and salary (Hoyt, 1974; Katz, 1973; Tuckman, Gapinski, & Hagemann, 1977).

Not only are tenure, promotion, salary, and the obtaining of grants important influences that motivate research and create stress, there are other factors and higher level needs that may exert a significant influence. It has been suggested that our collegial self-esteem depends on publishing (Aronson, 1981) and that fraud may be committed occasionally to obtain status and recognition (Garfield, 1987). There is some empirical evidence for these observations. In their factor analysis of a 45-item stress index that was completed by nearly 2000 faculty, Gmelch et al. (1986) reported that recognition was one of the factors that emerged. In a sample of academic and applied psychologists, Boice and Myers (1987) reported that 33% of the academic sample, compared with 5% of the private practice sampled, indicated lack of professional recognition as a source of stress.

In summary, it would appear that many sources of pressure in an academic setting concern the implementation of research. Some of the more obvious include promotion, tenure, salary, and likelihood of obtaining a grant and keeping the grant. Other sources of pressure, however, apparently contribute to stress concerning research productivity among academic faculty. These include the individual's uncertainty about how his or her research is evaluated and whether it is objectively evaluated, conflicts about how to use sparse time in carrying out teaching duties versus research duties, and the psychological importance of being valued and recognized by peers. In addition to all these factors, it appears to be increasingly difficult to publish research findings, given the high rejection rates, especially in prestigious journals. Any of these stressful circumstances could contribute to an individual scientist's committing research fraud.

FUTURE DIRECTIONS

This section will be organized along two themes. Most researchers who have addressed future directions in regard to handling academic dishonesty, fraud, or misrepresentation have advocated increased institutional involvement (e.g., committees to oversee various aspects of research integrity). This concept has been referred to as increasing policing mechanisms (Steneck, 1984). An overview of these suggestions will be presented first.

However, a different focus (i.e., often called prevention; Steneck, 1984) could be espoused that advocates a more personal and problem-solving approach before misconduct occurs. The second section will lay out these possibilities. If academic pressures contribute to incidents of fraud or misconduct, both of these foci should be in place to deal with the inherent contingencies in the system.

Policing Mechanisms

Policing mechanisms follow two lines: the establishment of formal policies for research ethics and the swift investigation of reports of fraud or misconduct. The establishment of policies for research ethics is clearly an educative approach. The following excerpt was taken from the University of Michigan Joint Task Force on Integrity of Scholarship and cited by Steneck (1984): "We hope to make clearer not only the types of integrity that are expected, but the contexts in which this integrity applies and should be judged" (p. 8). By having these principles in place, the institution and administration espouse guidelines for researchers that make clear, not only the ethical principles involved in conducting research, but also the institution's commitment to informing investigators of the appropriate conduct of experiments. Several examples follow.

Researchers need to be informed of the clear policies for retaining data or original records (Engler et al., 1987). Perhaps institutions should go so far as to inform investigators that data may need to be turned over to an appropriate committee for review, should allegations of misconduct surface. Mishkin (1988) suggested, "As a matter of institutional policy, the inability to provide primary data should give rise to a presumption that data do not (and never did) exist" (p. 1933). (However, as Braunwald, [1987], noted, Harvard had a clear policy to retain data and John Darsee did not comply.)

In addition, Mishkin (1988) and Engler et al. (1987) suggested that junior scientists should be supervised. Supervision should include "regular and systematic scrutiny of primary data, in-depth discussion of the analysis of the data, and continuing close personal interaction. There also should be instruction—through both expression and example—about respect for the data, wherever they may lead" (Mishkin, 1988, p. 1933).

A final policy that could be in place would govern the authorship of scientific articles. Several national organizations have such policies, including the American Psychological Association and the International Committee of Medical Journal Editors.

However, the institution will need to go at least one step further than the preceding guidelines. Various governmental agencies (e.g., NIH) now require that institutions have misconduct policies in place before grants or contracts are awarded (Powledge, 1986). Petersdorf

(1989) suggested that the guidelines issued by the Association of American Medical Colleges (1982) should serve as a model:

> The institution should be able to institute a process of inquiry rapidly and to complete it thoroughly, carefully, fairly, and expeditiously in an atmosphere of total, or at least relative, confidentiality. If a full-scale investigation is warranted, the means for proceeding should be on the books, and the responsibility of the institution, along with the rights of the accuser and the accused, should be clearly understood. At this point, the granting agency, whether public or private, should be informed that an investigation is in progress, but research funding should not be withdrawn until those conducting the investigation conclude that withdrawal is warranted, even though such delay may require the institution at which fraud has been committed to make retrospective restitution. (p. 121)

Finally, some researchers have advocated an atmosphere where the sanctions for confirmed reports of fraud or misconduct are clearly understood (Mishkin, 1988). Sanctions most often only come in the form of "loss of job or reputation . . . because of ignorance of the law or fear of the expense of litigation" (DuBois, 1989, p. 607). However, DuBois (1989) warned that the legal climate is changing and several individuals have been successfully convicted of crimes related to fraud.

To close, Mishkin (1988) suggested that the preceding policies should be incorporated "into student and faculty handbooks along with a statement that students and faculty are expected to be familiar with them and that major deviations are presumed to be intentional" (p. 1933). Also, she suggested that the policies be reviewed with students in laboratory courses. Mishkin (1988) provides an excellent overview of the process of responding to misconduct.

Prevention

A great deal of the preceding discussion could have been included in this section. The section on policing mechanisms, however, represents the institution's involvement in the process, and the following discussion will deal primarily with researchers per se.

The earlier discussion suggested personality variables and environmental contingencies that may play a role in leading an investigator to commit fraud or misconduct. Future research and practice should be aimed at addressing these potential mediators to decrease the probability of future occurrences of the questionable behavior.

Several authors have suggested that increased attention should be devoted to ethics training in the research community. An open and systematic discussion of ethics, research design, and so on, and routine inclusion of these issues in publications should help to increase awareness of the issues (DuBois, 1989). Braunwald (1987) also suggested, "It must be understood by all that to be a scientist is a privilege and that society invests a special trust in all scientists. Whenever that trust is abused it diminishes all scientists" (p. 216).

A second area to be revitalized is in the promotion of mentoring efforts. Woolf (1981) suggested that each individual scientist's "internal monitor [is learned from] mentors whose rigor and deliberate care guards them against wishful thinking and self-deception. This socialization is an essential component of professional education" (p. 11). This suggestion fits well with the earlier "institutional" requirement of providing supervision for junior scientists.

Another type of contact with other scientists would be to increase collaborative efforts. Woolf (1981) noted:

Research is highly interdependent; scientists communicate with each other at every stage in the process of investigation. From the inception of an idea for an experiment, to the development of protocols for carrying it out, to interpretation of results and preparation of a manuscript for publication, scientists are in touch with each other, testing their perceptions, ideas, and plans against those of colleagues. (p. 11)

Scientists would feel not only supported in their research efforts but also comfortable seeking out advice on problem issues. Collaborators could check data, computer printouts, graphs, or other research materials for each other (Petersdorf, 1986). Coauthors would also feel more comfortable with the data that are ultimately published. Blakely et al. (1986) suggested that "anyone willing to take credit for data collected by another must be equally willing to share the blame should those data prove fabricated" (p. 327).

In a somewhat different vein, administrators (and specifically chairs of departments) should be more involved in understanding the job strain involved in academic careers (Blackburn, Horowitz,

Edington, & Klos, 1986) and work with faculty to address concerns
and facilitate change in the inherent pressure and competition of the
job. Individuals who are making promotion and tenure decisions
should be more concerned with quality rather than with quantity of
research (Steneck, 1984). Angell (1986) suggested limiting the number
of publications that are considered for promotion or funding. She
suggested three probable effects of this change.

> First, the quality of medical research would tend to improve, insofar as
> each study would receive commensurately more attention. Second,
> promotions and funding would more accurately reflect the quality of a
> researcher's work, because a smaller number of publications would be
> easier to evaluate. Third, some of the fluff in our huge scientific litera-
> ture would be eliminated. (p. 262)

Angell (1986) and Bobys (1983) have also suggested that more
weight should be placed on excellence in teaching as a criterion for
promotion and tenure decisions. This may "reduce the push for publication that may lead to research fraud" (Bobys, 1983, p. 47).

Finally, administrators might direct special efforts toward burnout
prevention and intervention on faculty development (Dailey &
Jeffress, 1983), helping faculty to reduce Type A behaviors (Thurman,
1984, 1985) or restructuring faculty roles to decrease stress (Shull,
1972). This emphasis would be placed on the environmental contingencies that may contribute to fraudulent behavior.

CONCLUSIONS

A number of individuals have suggested that the process of sub-
mitting, reviewing, and accepting manuscripts for publication in professional journals should be changed to address some of the issues
raised in this chapter. Woolf (1981) suggested that all editors should
require authors to sign a statement that data will be available for 5
years postpublication. Relman (1989) suggested that editors ask
coauthors to accept responsibility for the integrity of studies that have
been submitted for publication, and Huth (1986) suggested that a
footnote include the exact contribution of each author. Engler et al.
(1987) believed that tables of data should be submitted to reviewers,

even if they are not to be part of the publication, so that reviewers would have more information to assess the representativeness of the data. Huth (1986) has also suggested that authors should be required to affirm that the "essence" of a manuscript has not been accepted for publication or already published elsewhere.

A number of authors have suggested that the scientific endeavor is both self-evaluative as well as self-correcting by nature of the replication of studies. However, during the past two decades, the publication of replications has become rare. Indeed, Engler et al. (1987) noted:

Replication, once an important element in science, is no longer an effective deterrent to fraud because the modern biomedical research system is structured to prevent replication—not to ensure it. It appears to be impossible to obtain funding for studies that are largely duplicative. (p. 1385)

Weinstein (1979) also noted that "the absence of and barriers to replication" (p. 650) is a real problem in the exacerbation of potentially fraudulent work because this self-policing mechanism is absent. Perhaps editors and grant institutions should be more willing to support replication studies.

A number of suggestions have been raised in considering the future directions that we can make to prevent or appropriately deal with fraud or instances of misconduct. DuBois's (1989) comments are quite cogent in the future assessment and treatment of the problem:

With respect to ethical conduct in research and the reporting thereof, what is required is deliberate effort on the part of scientific and professional organizations to define terms, to consider not a narrower but a wider range of problematic ethical situations, and to determine actual practices as opposed to accepted practices. (p. 611)

REFERENCES

Altman, L., & Melcher, L. (1983). Fraud in science. *British Medical Journal,* *286,* 2003–2006.

Angell, M. (1986). Publish or perish: A proposal. *Annals of Internal Medicine, 104,* 261–262.

Aronson, E. (1981). Research in social psychology as a leap of faith. In

E. Aronson (Ed.), *Readings about the social animal* (pp. 3–9). San Francisco: Freeman.

Association of American Medical Colleges. (1982). *The maintenance of high ethical standards in the conduct of research.* Washington, DC: Author.

Barrett, P. M. (1985, May). The premed machine. *The Washington Monthly,* 41–51.

Begley, S., Hager, M., & Doherty, S. (1987, February). Tempests in a test tube. *Newsweek,* 64.

Blackburn, R. T., Horowitz, S. M., Edington, D. W., & Klos, D. M. (1986). University faculty and administrator responses to job strains. *Research in Higher Education, 25,* 31–41.

Blakely, E., Poling, A., & Cross, J. (1986). Fraud, fakery, and fudging. In A. Poling & R. W. Fuqua (Eds.), *Research methods in applied behavior analysis* (pp. 313–330). New York: Plenum Press.

Bobys, R. S. (1983). Research fraud factors and effects. *Free Inquiry in Creative Sociology, 11,* 44–48.

Boice, R., & Myers, P. E. (1987). Which setting is healthier and happier, academe or private practice? *Professional Psychology: Research and Practice, 18,* 526–529.

Bornstein, M. H. (1980). Publication rates among distinguished American psychologists. *Bulletin of the British Psychological Society, 33,* 424.

Braunwald, E. (1987). On analysing scientific fraud. *Nature, 325,* 215–216.

Broad, W., & Wade, N. (1982). *Betrayers of the truth: Fraud and deceit in the halls of science.* New York: Simon and Schuster.

Brown, R. D., Bond, S., Gerndt, J., Krager, L., Krantz, B., Lukin, M., & Prentice, D. (1986). Stress on campus: An interactional perspective. *Research in Higher Education, 24,* 97–112.

Caplo, T., & McGee, R. J. (1965). How performance is evaluated. *The academic marketplace* (pp. 69–71). New York: Anchor Books.

Cicchetti, D. V., & Conn, H. O. (1976). A statistical analysis of reviewer agreement and bias in evaluating medical abstracts. *Yale Journal of Biology and Medicine, 49,* 373–383.

Cole, S., Cole, J. R., & Simon, G. A. (1981). Chance and consensus in peer review. *Science, 214,* 881–886.

Dailey, A. L., & Jeffress, C. A. (1983). Burnout prevention and intervention: Rationale and institutional strategies. *The Journal of College & University Personnel Association, 34,* 15–21.

DuBois, B. L. (1989). Accepted practices? A view from outside. *Perspectives in Biology and Medicine, 32,* 605–612.

Engler, R. L., Covell, J. W., Friedman, P. J., Kitcher, P. S., & Peters, R. M. (1987). Misrepresentation and responsibility in medical research. *The New England Journal of Medicine, 317,* 1383–1389.

Follette, V., & Klesges, R. C. (1988). Academic employment: A longitudinal study of the recruiting process and hired applicants. *Professional Psychology: Research and Practice, 19,* 345–348.

Fox, R. (1977). The medicalization and demedicalization of American society. *Daedalus, 106,* 9–22.

Frazier, P., Morrow, K., & Thoreson, R. (1990). *Work stress among male and female faculty members.* Unpublished manuscript.

Garfield, E. (1980). *The ethics of scientific publication. Essays of an information scientist.* Philadelphia: ISI Press.

Garfield, E. (1987). What do we know about fraud and other forms of intellectual dishonesty in science? Part 1. The spectrum of deviant behavior in science. *Current Comments, 14,* 3–7.

Gmelch, W. H., Lovrich, N. P., & Wilke, P. K. (1984). Sources of stress in academe: A national perspective. *Research in Higher Education, 20,* 477–490.

Gmelch, W. H., Wilke, P. K., & Lovrich, N. P. (1986). Dimensions of stress among university faculty: Factor-analytic results from a national study. *Research in Higher Education, 24,* 266–286.

Gottfredson, S. D. (1978). Evaluating psychological research reports. Dimensions, reliability, and correlates of quality judgments. *American Psychologist, 33,* 920–934.

Harrobin, D. F. (1989). The grants game. *Nature, 339,* 654.

Horowitz, S. M., Blackburn, R. T., Edington, D. W., & Kloss, D. M. (1988). Association between job stress and perceived quality of life. *Journal of American College Health, 37,* 29–35.

Hoyt, D. P. (1974). Interrelationships among instructional effectiveness, publication record, and monetary reward. *Research in Higher Education, 2,* 81–88.

Hunter, M. S., Ventimiglia, J., & Crow, M. L. (1980). Faculty morale in higher education. *Journal of Teacher Education, 31,* 27–30.

Huth, E. J. (1986). Irresponsible authorship and wasteful publication. *Annals of Internal Medicine, 104,* 257–259.

Katz, D. A. (1973). Faculty salaries, promotions, and productivity at a large university. *The American Economic Review, 63,* 469–477.

King, D. W., McDonald, D. D., & Roderer, N. K. (1981). *Scientific journals in the United States.* Stroudsburg, PA: Hutchinson Ross Publishing Co.

Knight, J. A. (1984). Exploring the compromise of ethical principles in science. *Perspectives in Biology and Medicine, 27,* 432–442.

Koshland, D. E. (1987). Fraud in science. *Science, 235,* 141.

Mahoney, M. J. (1976). *Scientist as subject: The psychological imperative.* Cambridge, MA: Ballinger Publishing.

Mahoney, M. J. (1979). Psychology of the scientist: An evaluative review. *Social Studies of Science, 9,* 349–375.

Merton, R. K. (1957). Priorities in scientific discovery: A chapter in the sociology of science. *American Sociological Review, 22,* 635–659.

Miers, M. L. (1985). Current NIH perspectives on misconduct in science. *American Psychologist, 40,* 831–835.

Miller, A. C., & Servan, S. L. (1984). Criteria for identifying a referred journal. *Journal of Higher Education, 55,* 673–697.

Mishkin, B. (1988). Responding to scientific misconduct due process and prevention. *Journal of the American Medical Association, 260,* 1932–1936.

Mullins, C. J. (1977). *A guide to writing and publishing in the social and behavioral sciences.* New York: Wiley.

Petersdorf, R. G. (1986). The pathogenesis of fraud in medical science. *Annals of Internal Medicine, 104,* 252–254.

Petersdorf, R. G. (1989, March). A matter of integrity. *Academic Medicine, 64,* 119–123.

Powledge, T. M. (1986, December). NIH Raub on misconduct. *The Scientist,* 18–19.

Relman, A. S. (1989, April). Fraud in science: Causes and remedies. *Scientific American, 260,* 126.

Rensberger, B. (1977, January). Fraud in research is a rising problem in science. *New York Times,* pp. 1, 44.

Scott, W. A. (1974). Interreferee agreement on some characteristics of manuscripts submitted to the *Journal of Personality and Social Psychology. American Psychologist, 29,* 698–702.

Seiler, R. E., & Pearson, D. A. (1984). Stress among accounting educators in the United States. *Research in Higher Education, 21,* 301–316.

Shukla, A., & Upadhyaya, S. B. (1986). Similar jobs: Dissimilar evaluations. *Psychologia, 29,* 229–234.

Shull, F. A., Jr. (1972). Professorial stress as a variable in structuring faculty roles. *Educational Administration Quarterly, 8,* 49–66.

Silver, G. A. (1983). The flower of medical science. *The Lancet, 2,* 332–333.

Steneck, N. H. (1984). Commentary: The university and research ethics. *Science, Technology, & Human Values, 9,* 6–15.

Stumpf, S. A., & Rabinowitz, S. (1981). Career stage as a moderator of performance relationships with facets of job satisfaction and role perceptions. *Journal of Vocational Behavior, 18,* 202–218.

Szilagyi, D. E. (1984). The elusive target: Truth in scientific reporting. *Journal of Vascular Surgery, 1,* 243–253.

Thurman, C. W. (1984). Cognitive-behavioral interventions with Type A faculty. *The Personnel and Guidance Journal, 62,* 277–278.

Thurman, C. W. (1985). Effectiveness of cognitive-behavioral treatments in reducing Type A behavior among university faculty—one year later. *Journal of Counseling Psychology, 32,* 445–448.

Tuckman, H. P., Gapinski, J. H., & Hagemann, R. P. (1977). Faculty skills and the salary structure in academe: A market perspective. *The American Economic Review, 67,* 692–702.

Weinstein, D. (1979). Fraud in science. *Social Science Quarterly, 59,* 639–652.

Willie, R., & Stecklein, J. E. (1982). A three-decade comparison of college faculty characteristics, satisfactions, activities, and attitudes. *Research in Higher Education, 16,* 81–93.

Wheeler, A. G. (1989). Publication pressures and disreputable behavior. *The Medical Journal of Australia, 150,* 464.

Woolf, P. (1981). Fraud in science: How much, how serious? *The Hastings Center Report, 11,* 9–14.

Woolf, P. K. (1986). Pressure to publish and fraud in science. *Annals of Internal Medicine, 104,* 254–256.

Zuckerman, H. (1977). Deviant behavior and social control in science. In E. Sagarin (Ed.), *Deviance and social change* (pp. 87–138). Beverly Hills, CA: Sage.

Zuckerman, H., & Merton, R. K. (1971). Patterns of evaluation in science: Institutionalization, structure, and functions of the referee system. *Minerva, 9,* 66–100.

CHAPTER 10

Editorial Processes, Safeguards, and Remedies

DANIEL X. FREEDMAN, MD

INTRODUCTION

The manifest potential of the life sciences has never been more exhilarating. But fraud, the unwelcome guest, perturbs our central focus on sound knowledge gain. All struggle for a sense of proportion, asking how much, why, where—in paleontology, chemistry, clinical trials, biomedicine, psychology—and what to do (Angell, 1988; Sharp, 1991). Further, the few blatant cases have ballooned into imputations of self-serving rather than science-serving conduct, possibly corrupting the entire endeavor of science. It is, in fact, an ill-defined situation and response seems awkward. Clearly, a disciplined and searching skepticism in critiquing scientific evidence is not an adequate preparation for the almost infinite regress of assessing malevolent personal motives and conduct and their varied socioenvironmental contexts. Nevertheless, a realistic review and updating of the expectations, practices, and arrangements for generating and communicating sound new knowledge offers promise that perspective can ensue.

THE RESPONSE OF THE EDITORIAL COMMUNITY

Editors, therefore, have been revisiting their procedures and their role in detecting fraud and acting on it (Angell, 1988; Huth, 1988; *JAMA*, 1990; Lundberg & Flanagin, 1989; Sharp, 1991). Other concerns—abuses of the editorial process by authors (Hanke et al., 1990)—entail a range of issues embracing self-serving activities that are wasteful of collegial resources or preempt the requirements of science. Plagiarism is easily defined (though not its motives). Now a new crime—self plagiarism—has arisen. Thus prolific yet honest authors, having tossed their goosequills to embrace their word processors' mindless memory of a rampant array of prose, are also in peril. They may awake to find their imperishable paragraphs doing dubious double duty in print. They thereby risk an ominous return of their abandoned goose!

Material that is unacknowledgedly essentially duplicative is now linked to "careerist abuses" of journals. Corrective procedures are under intensive review. When and why, for example, to publish an informative (but intrinsically admonitory or chastising) "Notice of Duplicate Publication" is a topic (Fulginiti, 1985; Hanke et al., 1990). The definitions of retraction, errata, corrections, corrections-and-amplifications, and the obligations of journals, academics, universities, research organizations, and government agencies with respect to journals and vice versa are other topics as yet less amplified—I will comment on them later.

Journals have, thus, increased precise requirements for authorial disclosures. Their major motive is to play their part in the implicit standard-setting and "modeling" of our aspirations for excellence that publications inevitably display. A concern for any "appearance" of a vested personal interest is also a driving factor. Of course, responsible scientists (and, incidentally, psychotherapists) systematically identify and explicitly deal with sources of personal interest and bias. This discipline, if practiced in the tiers of activity, from pre- and postdoctorals to their mighty laboratory chiefs and lofty institutional review committees, would surely be salutary.

Yet, the focus on appearances is generally on monetary interests, even though in that odd community called *Science* the "3 Ps" (priority, prestige, and publicity) are by far the more difficult interests to manage. Authors, in any event, now find they must sign extensive formalistic documents. There have been useful conferences and a growing literature, but also an almost bureaucratic editorial impulse to codify procedures. Definitions of authorship, of the permitted numbers of authors, of undesirable "honorary authorship" and even of what is to be signified by the order of authorship (Riesenberg & Lundberg, 1990) have also been broached.

The vanity of editors and journals that "have been took" is injured, but, with some exceptions, constructive action has ensued. Lundberg et al. justifying the move to increased documentary requirements of authors, well state a widely perceived need by editors (*JAMA*, 1989):

> To educate authors and help them avoid the pitfalls of ignorance and to discourage a few from believing that ethics and laws do not apply to them, peer-reviewed journals codify their policies and procedures in Instructions for Authors. . . . However, pressures to publish, increased competition in the research and academic communities, and inadequate education of researchers and authors have allowed naive authors to unknowingly transgress the ill-defined boundaries of publication and authorial ethics, and a lack of formal policies (or enforcement thereof) has allowed dishonest authors to intentionally deceive." (p. 2003)

Some weakly motivated deceivers might be discouraged by formal "policies." It would, however, be naive and a failure to grasp the social psychology of the con artist, to believe that pronouncements, oaths, and signatures really accord the science community immunity from fraud. Education of the community generating research is, indeed, needed and, in fact, overdue. The post-World War II explosion of knowledge spurred laboratories, technology, personnel, and funding in our institutions, which grew like Topsy. All elements could benefit by a pause to catch up with overall principles (and their purpose) that guide comportment in scientific endeavor.

The Problems of Overreacting

With respect to what editors and journals can and should do in the service of remediation, I have an underlying concern that our reforms may inadvertently symbolically contribute to a larger uncollegial and fundamentally antiscientific atmosphere. Woebetide today's scientist who miscalculates a statistic or produces an error in print, or who in good faith trusts colleagues or computer printouts of complex clinical research. For the contemporary environment is one in which, even simple, unintended and candidly recognized mistakes can connote mischief and malevolence. Thus, from imprecise media news (and the gossip dignified as "news departments" in leading journals) most of us gain our notions about questioned scientific conduct. Where there is a problem or dispute, few examine the complex primary data and only exceptionally distinguished reporters are both comprehensive and precise. Overly trusting scientists who are victims of complexity and error thereby suffer "amputation of reputation" by loosely defined criteria on conduct that is often inexpertly assessed by defensive or uninstructed official review bodies, without the semblance of due process. Congressional hearings ("guerrilla theatre") heighten the milieu of mistrust (Angell, 1988). As has been sardonically quipped, "Ask not for whom the science conduct bell tolls—it Dingles for all un-Weiss enough to publish new knowledge!"

In the long history of theological reformations of conduct and belief, a radical sanctimonious pietism has been as corruptive of the fundamental missions of revered institutions as the poor practices that evoked the reform. Thus, the envisioned role of editors in scrutinizing the bank accounts and laboratory notebooks of contributors not only is hardly feasible but is probably inappropriate. Nor is discourse precise in distinguishing between innovative clinical investigation and "hired hands" producing routine data and the wide array of disparate documents requisite for new drug applications. The judgment of the Food and Drug Administration's (FDA) former sardine factory inspectors or fiscal auditors on scientifically significant or trivial documentary lapses have been used to characterize current clinical science as a whole. In response, journals have been urged to rescue the entirety of science by dispatching Sir Galahads to "randomly audit" laboratory practices (as does the FDA). To be precise, for the collegium of clinical research experts and their academic societies *and* institutions some would substitute editors to *sponsor* random audits of clinical research (Rennie, 1989). This represents an extreme overreaching of editorial roles, services, and accountabilities.

Full Disclosure as a Corrective Action

The preceding remarks bear on gaining perspective on safeguards and remedies in the editorial process for fraud (and the different domain of poor practices). It is necessary first to define the purpose of journals. In our rightful concern about problematic reports, we may forget the underlying "guiding principles" of what journals are all about. What will follow, then, derives from 20 (thoroughly enjoyable) years of editing the *Archives of General Psychiatry*. If editors do not run the world, it may also be useful to gain perspective on what the actual ambit of editorial accountability realistically comprises.

I summarize general guiding principles as *full disclosure,* and I do so without imposing minutely detailed codifications. The latter can become pro forma expressions of "Sundays only" duty rather than faithful manifestations of good works stemming from belief! Full disclosure (Freedman, 1988a), as I will later amplify, describes adequately what is truly within the province of editors and the obligations of all in transactions with them (including institutions and agencies—or occasionally even advertisers). I will draw extensively on my editorials (Freedman, 1982; Freedman, 1988a), to which authors are, in fact, referred in "Instructions to Authors." I reproduce a part of our current Instructions to demonstrate the tone and principles of what we expect and what we expect as a condition to consider an article.

> The collegiality of reliable science communications entails full, open exchange of information about a report and its history. . . . Authors' identification of special circumstances, vested interests, or sources of bias that might be deemed to affect the integrity of the reported information is requisite. . . . (For) any questions about . . . possible duplicative material, or other special circumstances . . . the editor will gladly confer. . . .
>
> Readers . . . (need) . . . sufficient data to arrive at their own informed assessments . . . (and can) . . . be informed of the history, divisions of labor, or special circumstances of a report within the published text and

with the identification of affiliations and full acknowledgments of aid, advice and support.

Authorship does not claim expertise in every aspect of the work. It does mean that each author within his or her own limits has exerted sufficient reasonable effort to vouch for the validity of the entire work and to bear public accountability for maintaining the integrity of the scientific information communicated. Each author must have had enough substantial involvement in generating and formulating the published product to bear such accountability.

And in conveying the copyright to us, all authors sign a statement that:

I have been sufficiently involved in this work to take public responsibility for its validity and final presentation as an original publication. I can provide documentation of my work upon reasonable request and I have fulfilled the obligations for full disclosure and authorship as described by *Archives of General Psychiatry*.

Taken seriously, the spirit and readiness to practice full disclosure for peer review captures most of the safeguards and remedies that are within the province of authors and journals to implement on behalf of the integrity of science reports (Freedman, 1988a).

EDITORIAL PROCESSES AND SYSTEMS—THEIR PURPOSE AND PROCEDURES

Scientific journals have a unique position in the network of enterprises comprising the social system called science. Their primary function is to mediate the needs of authors, referees, and readers for sound scientific communications, and to do so with vigilant regard for scholarly and scientific standards. Although this serves the broader societal interests in sound knowledge, journals centrally relate to select universes of directly interested parties. However journals are situated, whatever their particular aims, funding, or sponsorship, they share in the uncodified but broadly accepted standards of all the systems of science.

Thus, peers in science address peers with information—available to all who would peer into a journal's pages. Whatever its relative value, that information is expected to be essentially authentic. As noted elsewhere (Freedman, 1988a):

> . . . observations presented in a form that can be assessed by journal referees, editors and readers provide more than information. Information becomes useful knowledge if it can be critiqued and further tested in both systematic study and clinical practice as well as reflected on in order to sharpen and enlarge professional perspectives. (p. 690)

This is at the heart of the editorial purpose in mediating scientific communications.

The contributions to evolving knowledge—the published products—represent the efforts of both contributors and the editorial process. Authors, each and all, are the primary agents with whom journals customarily deal. Occasionally the National Academy of Sciences or other related agencies form committees to oversee or communicate published research, but institutional sponsorship for authorship is rarely the case. With the increasingly common complex or multisite collaborative research projects, a rapporteur or a guiding committee can be the effective transmitter of reports and may appear on the authorial by-line. Credibility of such reports rests on their content and on the full assent of the accountable collaborators (Freedman, 1982). Personal credit need not thereby be vitiated, although prominence is.

Essentially, however, it is authors who publicly vouch to their peers who review, edit, and publish their work for the contribution that bears their names. Theirs is the "signature of authenticity." The editorial processes cannot and do not ultimately vouch for this. Rather, the editorial process assumes authenticity and mediates prior and subsequent critical discourse about a product whose quality as a publication is judged for a complex of needs and "trusts" (Lundberg & Flanagin, 1989).

In the act of publishing, the journal publicly asserts its belief that the authors' information is in a format, and is sufficiently informative and sound in content and interpretation, to share with readers. Readers, in turn, bear accountability for arriving at their own assessment of the report and editorial judgments. Dyspeptic editors have a special vantage from which to arrive at a dismal opinion of the "scientific literacy" of authors and readers—indeed in the ability or willingness of audiences to read what is precisely said and what is *not* claimed. The soundness of science rests on the fact that its conclusions, whatever the important problems addressed, are intrinsically tightly limited by the constraints of method and designs. Thus, unwarranted conclusory assertions can be edited; editorial comment can be published; but the *inferences* readers draw are in the head of the perceiver. There comes a point after energetic editorial and authorial struggling for clarity and ethical concern for possible misinterpretations, where, for the consumer, *caveat emptor* must rule.

In the review process, the editor selects experts for critique of methodology, scholarship, interpretations, expository clarity, and importance in the topic area. These actions generate colloquy and exchange. Strikingly, this is a voluntary exercise. The unpaid collegium who submit and others who tirelessly review are powerful testimony to the values and belief system of science. Error, gross oversight, bias, and envy, along with sharp and helpful observations and argument characterize the responses to submissions. Authors in my experience are most often grateful for the helpful parts of these unpaid consultations, even though they often mindlessly burden colleagues with grossly insufficient presubmission scrutiny.

The editor, using advice from colleagues and the editorial board, must finally evaluate the entire review process—"diagnose" it for both substantive merits and sources of bias. Ultimately, the editor decides on the adequacy and fairness of advice and, then, on the suitability of the product in terms of the journal's aims and mission.

The entire process does not comprise a final Jovian judgment on the ultimate or enduring value of the contribution. (Such hubris may be harbored but should not be indulged.) That order of judgment is intrinsically impossible in the evolving and self-corrective system of science. Further, the annual proliferation of new journals hardly prevents unappreciated genius from seeing print. When publication is the final verdict, the journal simply asserts that in conformity with its mission this product is now considered worth sharing in the service of science.

In all this, there is the essential trust that the integrity of the intent and processes of producing the information are not at issue. Questions regularly arise during the review process that bear on design, execution, methods, precision, analyses, scholarship, and quality of the study. These questions might (or might not) bear on integrity. But at this early juncture of review, trust in the intention of honest reportage prevails. So, as I remarked of the finally published product; ". . . the mere perception of errors, oversights, contradictions, poor choice of analytic methods and flaws" does not undermine the fundamental trust in the authors' integrity in reporting what they have done. Such flaws are to be expected. Rather ". . . it is their collegial ascertainment that is integral to the way that science works. Opportunity for their detection is what journals and the review process systematically intend to provide. . . ." (Freedman, 1988a, p. 690).

Thus, this process does provide the safeguards of earnest but intrinsically imperfect scrutiny, critique, and discussion prior to publication that, in turn, should provoke more thought and comments. Where issues are in dispute at the *Archives of General Psychiatry,* we have always insisted—or at least wistfully hoped—that the grounds for dispute be clarified and, where possible, the next steps for resolution of dispute (or puzzles) be identified. We usually insist on this *prior* to publication of an article. We may not publish when authors refuse to recognize that a telephone call to a colleague or provision to readers of alternative explanations may prevent several years of printed argument. There are times when technical experts should first convene in person to resolve arcane or picayune dispute.

For journals, the status of the substantive science issues and the form of their communication have primacy. The comportment of scientists is usually not directly relevant. Sound science reports come from a variety of persons and from some with undesirable traits along the entire range from unpleasant to thoroughly noxious behaviors, but still not conduct that corrupts the integrity of information reported. Sloppy science can see print. It represents poor judgment of authors and in the review process. It is hoped that these are a lapse rather than habit. The sanctions for it, however, should not be viewed as being in the same category as the malevolent intent of "misconduct" and consequent mandatory obloquy. Habitual unreliability generates its own consequences. Sanctions for lapses in judgment ensue in the informal rankings and referrals within the life of the science communities, or in independent objective assessments of qualifications for the rewards of academic advancement. Contributors and journal subscriptions can "sanction" poor editorial habits.

All publication entails the exhibition of personal effort. Yet, publication of scientific information and opinion about it rests on an odd and exceptionally disciplined process even though both authors and journals are "showing their wares." In science we all—journals, institutions, and authors—traverse what I have called the "multi-mirrored corridors of vanity and envy." But we, almost uniquely, are to surrender self-interest, at least for the moment of review, on behalf of the integrity of scientific information. We submit ourselves not simply to argument but to the rigorous examination of our evidence (and intransigently cherished premises). All engage in an inexorable search for error.

Because editors are tempted to compete for the prizes of prestige or publicity, they should be alert to the pitfalls of hasty judgments in the quest for eminence. But even if our focus is modest and our allegiance as scientists to the intrinsic task is foremost, scientific groups have an urge and an inherent social need to hierarchically rank the repositories of their strivings. Thus authors ambivalently project a burden of flawless excellence and perception of authority on the "top journals." Their editors must then avoid the temptations of pomposity while enforcing the principle that all in the collegium are equal, as all submit to the gauntlet of evidentiary review and seek the sources of error to generate new knowledge. I have wondered, as instant electronic communication grows, whether journals will become obsolete. I doubt it, because there is (while I'm inventing "social instincts") an "archival" urge—a need to preserve the products of our effort in an accessible, retrievable, and enduringly recognizable, palpable form.

Thus for journals the "it"—the science communicated—and the authorial vouching for it and collegial but searching critique of it are, ideally, the central processes. In general, the product, far more than the personalities generating it or the interpersonal strivings entailed in its production, is at issue. And as the topic evolves through further colloquy and work, *the structure of knowledge with respect to the topic is what primarily is at stake.*

DETECTION OF FRAUD

Most would agree that trust in science is essential. Thus, in the very fabric of the generation and communication of scientific knowledge, concerned attention is directed to flaws in the production of information—to self-deceptions, but not to the contrived deception of others. Accessibility to data and critique of it are the "rules," providing valued checks and balances. These habits are at the heart of the folkways and customs that govern conduct in science. So skepticism, critique, a thoroughgoing inquisition of submitted or published material are in an entirely different realm from the search for culpability when uncivil breaches of other social mores, including criminal breaches, are the issues. Authors are *responsible* for error, for overlooking a possibility, and for succumbing to the common fault of the self-deceptions of wishful credulity. They are not thereby *culpable* or guilty of corruptive intent. Critics are vulnerable to similar flaws. Both are rescued as the scientific methods works its way. Nor, if the advance of knowledge is the goal, is poor scholarship a crime. "Useful discovery can be impeded by knowing too much . . . discovery does not require that working hypotheses be accurately based . . . (but) the test of discovery and a critically articulated knowledge base surely do!" (Freedman, 1987, p. 25). So, there is a common bond of trusted intent; critics and authors are assumed to be in pursuit of the construction of an ever sounder base of scientific knowledge.

The "mental set," in the editorial process is, then, not readily cued to detect fraud. The editor's desk surely sees submissions that are all too raw and in which the information disclosed is too jumbled to provide the fundamental basis for review and judgment. Editors see other serious flaws and unpleasant practices (Angell, 1983). As Hersen noted to me, we should be alert to material that is too good, or to being mesmerized by dazzling productivity that is implausibly prolific (personal communication, 1990). In my experience, one of the major recurrent questions is "What is the publication strategy of this scientist or laboratory or project?" Sound scientific journalism should itself be informed by some *plan* for reportage. Readers should know what is in the pipeline or being simultaneously analyzed and the like. So "fragmentation" in publication (the "least publishable unit") is viewed as a noxious practice—but not necessarily fraud.

Angell (1983) notes the problem of skewed selection of material from a data set. "Trimming" is an unsavory practice that referees often, but not always, detect. But selective omissions to strengthen a report may or may not represent fraud. More generally, it derives from a near delusional belief on the part of scientists in the hypothesis they are pursuing. They wish to compel the belief of others. To be more precise, in my experience as a reviewer and editor, such authors generally have a point that is interesting and sustainable but not *as* compelling as their personal belief. Such instances could signal possible deceptive practices requiring "notification," especially when, on editorial inquiry, the authors are unresponsive or provide improbable reply.

But the latter class of cases have not led us to eventual discovery of deliberate intent to deceive. They conceivably occasionally might if institutional cognizance and intent to scrutinize were pursued. More commonly, this is instigated by close colleagues, staff, or students as "whistle-blowers." Although some "selective submitters" have been judged by us as being not very credible, sufficient evidence to cause us confidently to identify "probable deception" as a problem has been encountered only once—and could not later be institutionally clearly validated.

With respect to less than optimal science reporting, journals add their own push to the widely noted pressures deriving from the funding or the academic survival sectors of the life of science. The compressed "sanitized" presentations of complex work that we require (with space constraints in mind) surely tempts the smoothing out of rougher realities. This can cumulatively be misleading if not deceptive. In the past decades of controlled clinical research we have unintentionally generated images of an "order of certitude" expected of publishable hypothesis-generating work that is sheerly unrealistic. A more faithful reflection in print of the honest but grueling quest for knowledge would provide a workable reflection of the state of the art and expectations of it.

Breuning in Retrospect

In reviewing our experience with the Breuning story (Freedman, 1988b), it is clear that the six referees and the correspondence during the subsequent 2 years of resubmission, focused on methods, analyses, and extensively on inferences. It is also explicit that I was struck and irritated by Breuning's lack of authentic grasp of the clinical pharmacology of neuroleptics and his lack of years of research experience with them, as well as by his gratuitous social policy or clinical practice advice (all of which was excised). Given the intensity of expert review, what, then, did we miss or could we have done that might have detected the fraud or prevented its publication?

I find two mental sets and one habit of journals and authors worth noting. Foremost is the fact that neither the locale nor time period in which Breuning's data were collected nor the different authorial functions were specified in the text. That habit (a derivative of sanitized and compressed reportage) of not providing, or *requiring,* such detail is ingrained and widespread. Reflection on that reinforces my insistence on good journalism: The *who, what, when, where, how,* and *why* of an inquiry must be reported.

In science we are essentially to tell the story of our work (Freedman, 1982, 1988a). Breuning not only "told a story," he produced a fictional work that caricatures what is entailed in complex research and that subtly exposes the flaws of the science community's lapsed standards for keeping accessible records, or for coauthors' insistence on accessing them. Had the detail been *explicitly* required and supplied, the result still might not have alerted us to a problem. But perhaps his coauthors, hospital staff, or university colleagues might have been alerted before or, at least, after publication.

This leads to the set of two comfortable assumptions that may, if recognized, help in implementing a more completely informed review. The extensive—on reflection, phenomenal—series of day-and-night observations he reported might have raised eyebrows. But our habit of uncritically assuming that there is "institutional awareness" of a study's detail and execution may have diverted query. We are lulled and gulled by our wishes, as every con artist well knows. The wishful assumption may have been that there was sponsorship from the top rank, richly research-intensive environment from which the piece was dispatched, thus diverting queries of plausibility. I, at least, in friendly but frankly expressed exasperation had finally referred Dr. Breuning for counsel to his university colleagues known by me to be clinically and pharmacologically trained experts with neuroleptic studies.

A second less relevant and perhaps more conscious mental set was that the study of mentally retarded children was a topic I thought ought, if possible, to be rescued. One purpose of the journal is to alert our readership to populations and topics or approaches in which we do not specialize but are of relevance to general psychiatry. The rarity of quality submissions on the topic and the fact that retardation was an area in which I had once dabbled (e.g., Schain & Freedman, 1961) could have caused more editorial patience—though not latitude—than normal. I cannot be certain.

That is the best I can do to examine in retrospect how we might have been less blind. I do not sufficiently know the mental and "value sets" of the six reviewers of the original submission to ascribe mine to them. But none of us—even with the best of reportage—could have detected fraud. Rather, inquiry conceivably might have been instigated that, in turn, might have done so. I finally should comment that I do not accept that the highly constrained report of a one-shot effort with a neuroleptic could have influenced practices by any adequately clinically trained medical practitioner. One must simply read the tightly explicit reservations that 2 years of tortured review required of any of Dr. Breuning's assertions. Thus, the article was finally published simply as a signal to the world of psychiatry and pharmacology that there was a population deserving of systematic study.

Prevention

Whether or not there is protection in our practice of often employing far more than two referees, the purpose in so doing has never been concern for fraud. Some find it forbidding and bewildering. A rare few loftily dismiss it as obviously unnecessary for them. But most find it enriches critique. I believe it helps sustain the standards and substance of the science with which we deal. The collegial intent is to provide authors with a useful "sampler of informed reader response" and to enable them, if possible, to provide sufficiently salient argument or detail within the text to reduce the necessity for subsequent published—and often narcissistically exhibitionist—"ping-pong." Such published colloquies consume chunks of our highly rationed monthly page allotments. And so in collegial intent, I instruct authors to "diagnose" how they are read rather than to endure the agony of grudgingly or ritually satisfying each of the points of each referee. I do not allow referees to dictate what authors have a right to defend and say, but rather urge authors to have their say after an opportunity for careful thought about the perceptions of others.

In any event, this wider net once clearly served to prevent rank plagiarism, which I've encountered but once in my 20 years. Two Boston experts, nationally eminent for their literate opining on the topic, found the piece passable. A third, more plebeian and with a plodding, scholarly bent, instantly supplied the evidence that the total document had been plagiarized. Because 20% or less of received submissions see print in *Archives,* we have no ultimate evidence as to what criminal mischief the multiple reviews and rejections, even though they did not detect fraud, may have missed or discouraged.

REMEDIES TO CORRECT THE LITERATURE

Many kinds of problems cross the editor's desk and must be dealt with on a case-by-case approach. There is little documented "case law," but rather considered commonsense to guide the process. Obviously, when journals err, errata are due. When nontrivial errors or problems with a report are known, it is the author's obligation ultimately to notify the journal and subsequently its readers; at that juncture coauthors are similarly accountable. A reader may raise questions; and the editor, as a "matchmaker," may arrange for authors and the reader to correspond. If the wider readership should be informed, discourse or comment (usually as Letters to the Editor) may follow. "Corrections" the authors offers can be published in Letters. Many are, in fact, quite extensive—usually instigated by discovery of a major mix-up (commonly generated by the distance from primary data that the mischievous convenience of computers enhances). "Corrections and Amplifications" are then published in the Letters Department. For these steps what is requisite for the science literature is that the *evolving "science story" be trackable.* Indexing services must be enabled to provide such information. When they can, the journal has done its job. Thereafter, a strong appetite for scholarship by other investigators (who are accountable for reviving the almost abandoned scholarly habit of searching the literature) becomes requisite.

Retraction, however, is an ill-defined step (Maddox, 1988). When does a "Correction and Amplification" become a retraction? Colaianni (National Library of Medicine, 1989), describing the actions of the literature-tracking services of MEDLINE and *Index Medicus,* notes that the occasions may range from pervasive error, irreproducible (add irretrievable) data, conclusions based on faulty logic or computations, data generated by accidental contamination or retrospectively discovered equipment flaws, to falsifications and fabrications. What, for purposes of tracking the literature, does the retraction say of the substance of science? If the latter is key, is it not possible, as has been done, to retract a portion but not all of a report? If words mean what dictionaries say rather than what editorial Humpty Dumptys claim, it should be possible to "withdraw statements" without prejudice. But the current trend of investigatory review bodies is to "prescribe retraction" as the severest of punishments—recantation and excommunication. Accordingly, the term has been viewed by some editors as synonymous with an unarguable judgment of fabricated or *totally* unworthy (rather than unworkable) evidence and untrustworthy authorship.

Yet the absence of available adequate records or the inadequacy of records or instruments on re-review to yield satisfactory information about matters in dispute may in fact be the case. It requires courage to assert that on such a basis certain conclusions must be "withdrawn." Where the effort and pain of patients and honest investigators have produced information—some or all of which must be withdrawn—it is, I believe, unethical and collegially inappropriate not to report in a "retraction" some considered comment on the status of the science problems originally addressed. So retraction, where fraud is *not* the issue, should be informative. The rubric should not connote more than notice of a substantive comment on the status of previously reported information and a notice that facilitates tracking of the literature. Retraction represents a judgment about the status of the science—not about the conduct of retractors.

Finally, who retracts? Depending on the situation, one or all authors may wish to be dissociated from a conclusion for a range of reasons. Essentially, as Lundberg once quipped "authors tract and must retract," and, I would add, the interested collegium "tracks." Journals cannot retract. They can "repudiate" their association with a piece (Freedman, 1988b), in effect, yield their copyright and notify the National Library of Medicine.

Where there is authorial reluctance to amplify, then what I call a "moral surrogate" must act to vouchsafe the integrity of science reporting. This generally entails the intervention of institutional resources with their capacity for investigative reviews. *Notification* to journals of problems and the implementing of steps for their correction by authors is the ideal. It is simply accomplished and, from my

vantage, has been ably done over the years with "Corrections and
Amplifications." Rarely, however, do coauthors grasp their role to
participate, to assent or dissent. A few editors—at some risk, I
believe—have simply published a "Notice of Retraction" without
soliciting authorial input and with naive total reliance on an outside
and unexamined "authoritative" judgment.

INSTITUTIONS AND JOURNALS

At the heart of editorial work is the sustained exercise of judgment.
When the labor of others can substitute for such decisions, it is
tempting to relax. It is also a lapse of editorial duty! Institutions have
their own agenda, prestige, and political pressures. In no "misconduct case" have I ever been informed of problems in a timely or
appropriate way by any academic or governmental institution, and I
have been thereby pragmatically impeded in instituting appropriate
prompt action. I should add that where public health urgency for hard
information exists—a correct drug dose or caution to "suspend action
until further notice," and so on—journals are *not* constrained. This
authentic urgency, however (perhaps unhappily so) is rarely the case
for us. Many solid research labors that we rightly publish, in terms of
their effect on evolving knowledge share an ineffable quality of time-
lessness.

Two examples of transactions with institutions come to mind. The
voluminous 1987 NIMH report on Breuning reflected the excellent
work of a truly top-notch panel. The bulky package was courteously
transmitted. But the arrogance of the Institute in also transmitting a
letter—deliberately not stipulated as publishable—and stating that
they "expected" the journal to ". . . take whatever steps are necessary to expunge the literature . . ." was hardly helpful. That steps *had*
previously been taken (and missed the cognizance of both the NIMH
staff and panel) is irrelevant. Generically, though, what "steps" does
an editor take? All that institutions can properly ask of a journal is that
we publish *their* opinion, but the Institute's was not offered in
publishable form. If an institution does request such publication, we
can then easily solicit the authors' opinions and finally render our own
judgment. Truly responsible journals do not totally surrender their
accountability to judge to any outside agency but do need their help.

I provided a lengthy account, under the rubric "Request for Retraction" (Freedman, 1988b), when we repudiated our association with the article. The intent was to document what a journal can and cannot do when authors do not agree on retraction (and we do hold *all* authors accountable for a response) as well as to detail how we arrived at a judgment. After several years of publicity, the judgment was not difficult—even though no institution had earlier directly alerted us. Yet, properly arraying the evidence for journal exposition was extraordinarily difficult. Lacking a precise communication and permission to publish, we had—for legal (and ethical) purposes—carefully and painstakingly to reconstruct our transactions and then abstract the essence of the problem simply to assert it correctly. Fortunately, the ADAMHA Administrator had publicly blurted his own concise assessment that we could quote, but the actual NIMH reviewing body would not oblige. We had then to extract current addresses of all authors from NIMH and proceed to elicit their responses.

As an exhaustive investigative report, the NIMH document was adequately formatted. But it is solely a particular *article* (not a complex set of them) that is initially at issue for a particular journal. The pragmatic problem in the final notifying of the journal was the *lack of precision in meeting our publication needs.* The rules for authors, in brief, should apply to agencies. In sum, the process was slowed because the steps of formatting a publishable and concise "notice" that serves a journal's purposes were simply not grasped. Finally, the report itself—though not Breuning, who explicitly raised the point—missed the accountability of *all* coauthors to access data and notify journals.

Similar obligations to notify journals concisely in publishable format, and recognition that all authors owe the journal information, rest with university reviews. In one egregious case, a coerced and excessively detailed notification—the fact of coercion and corporate "ghosting" of the document not disclosed—was received without copyright and with a request for advice on how to proceed to correct the literature. The request was answered in detail. The cordially invited next steps to guide a concise publishable letter, and advice to supply copyright for it, were never taken. The deception about the true authorship in the notification remained hidden. The journal was then scurrilously publicly attacked as being obstinately dilatory (and more), although the steps for efficient and prompt publication were simple and clear. Institutional guile, urgencies, and defensiveness are facts of life. Fortunately, the key authors were responsible—both to the journal and readers. They volunteered their own early notice of problems and when a letter was feasible, a timely and publishable focus on the substance of science. Strikingly, none of the institutional (including governmental) reviewing parties involved squarely addressed that subject. In this case, the university, in patent distortion of the meaning of the science entailed, quite late in the process even tried lamely to invent a "public health urgency" to what was, in uncontestable fact, a clinically irrelevant and recondite hypothesis-generating exercise in pathophysiology.

WHAT EDITORS AND AUTHORS CAN EASILY DO

When problems come across the editor's desk, about all that can be done is to gain the opinion and evaluation of peers or authors and coauthors by use of telephone, fax, or correspondence. *That* is the clear ambit or province of the editorial process. Occasionally, the editor must refer problems to others better situated to resolve them, but the usual first step is to continue the principles of the review process and colloquy among the involved parties and experts. I assume that authors have data available for review and that all members and leaders of research groups actively seek to be adequately informed and actively seek to inform others effectively. If the data are available for authorial or consultants' review, most problems can be identified and reported in print. Sheer deception, when it occurs—as it will—is unlikely seriously to derail the knowledge base, given the gauntlet of science's repeated scrutinies.

Full disclosure and unassuming good journalistic reportage reduce risks for all, including investigators. The complexity of modern science, divisions of labor, and computers can distance the scientific team from primary events. But know-how with respect to the personnel and the systems for assembling the primary research data, prudent record keeping, and a striving by each and all to be informed (rather than to take a passive spectator posture toward the arrival of data) can diminish misconstruals and error. The history of the problem, its current pursuit, and availability of all reports of commonly accessed material in the project's archival data banks can be a part of the research team's life. Prior agreements on divisions of labor and authorship can be explicitly arranged, and realistic definitions of expectations of the most junior and senior participants can be specified. These collegial practices—if we stem our current censorial obsessions to revenge lapses (usually with retroactively imposed standards)— can restore an environment in which collegial trust will be able to guide confident comportment in necessary divisions of labor.

THE JOURNALISTIC IDEAL

The underlying operating and safeguarding principle is fairly simple. Full disclosure means disclosing the essential details so that colleagues can track the "story" of a research endeavor and its evolution. This is why all of the furor about duplicate publication resolves in my view not only to wasted resources but simply to an obstruction of the ability of the science community readily to track the evolving science story.

So I have argued (Freedman, 1988a) and, in conclusion, repeat that authors have an obligation to "tell it as it happened." Some journal space to do so should be accommodated. A clear and sound journalistic report can be concise. The who, what, when, how, and why of a study permits authors credibly to share their experience—the ultimate purpose of all the labor of scientific communication. Readers can be enabled to visualize who the actual patients are and the culture of the settings encountering them (Kupfer & Freedman, 1986). This does not require exhaustive or obsessive detail because, even if needed for the review, such material can later be "available on request." There is absolutely no need to mask the problems in the real world of research. To the contrary. Any of us who know firsthand the disorderly realities of clinical and laboratory life can appreciate the real triumph represented by orderly analyses of it and the proper uses of design, methods, and controls for error. The structure of our solid knowledge base has thereby truly advanced by painstaking steps, commonly by convergent lines of evidence, and rarely by salient breakthrough (Freedman, 1987).

System Considerations and Safeguards

CONCLUSION

On reflection and review, I still believe—and not because of my perseverative defects—that trust is *not* an unaffordable luxury (Freedman, 1988a):

It requires an expenditure of effort—the constant, even painful, exercise of critical judgment. That, however, is a luxury we cannot afford *not* to implement. In brief, our ultimate purpose in the high risk of scientific endeavor and in full disclosure is not to catch a thief but rather to apprehend useful knowledge. (p. 691)

REFERENCES

Angell, M. (1983). Editors and fraud. *Council of Biology Editors Views, 6,* 3–8.

Angell, M. (1988). Fraud in biomedical research: A time for congressional constraint. *New England Journal of Medicine, 318,* 1462–1463.

Freedman, D. X. (1982). Megamultiple authorships. *Archives of General Psychiatry, 39,* 351.

Freedman, D. X. (1987). Strategies for research in biological psychiatry. In H. Y. Meltzer (Ed.), *Psychopharmacology: The Third Generation of Progress* (pp. 23–30). New York: Raven Press.

Freedman, D. X. (1988a). The meaning of full disclosure. *Archives of General Psychiatry, 45,* 689–691.

Freedman, D. X. (1988b). Request for retraction. *Archives of General Psychiatry, 45,* 685–686.

Fulginiti, V. A. (1985). Unfortunately, more on duplicate publication. *American Journal of the Diseases of Children, 139,* 865–866.

Hanke, C. W., Arndt, K. A., Dobson, R. L., Dzubow, L. M., Parish, L. C., & Taylor, J. S. (1990). Dual publication and manipulation of the editorial process. *Archives of Dermatology, 126*(12), 1625–1626.

Huth, E. J. (1988). Retraction of research findings. *Annals of Internal Medicine, 108,* 304.

Journal of the American Medical Association (JAMA) (1990). *263,* 1317–1438.

Kupfer, D. J., & Freedman, D. X. (1986). Treatment for depression: "Standard" clinical practice as an unexamined topic. *Archives of General Psychiatry, 43,* 509–511.

Lundberg, G. D., & Flanagin, A. (1989). New requirements for authors:

Signed statements of authorship responsibility and financial disclosure. *Journal of the American Medical Association, 262,* 2003–2004.

Maddox, J. (1988). How to say sorry graciously. *Nature, 433,* 13.

National Library of Medicine (1989). Errata, retraction and comment policy. *National Library of Medicine Fact Sheet June 1989.* Bethesda: National Institutes of Health, PHS, USDHHS.

Rennie, D. (1989). Editors and auditors. *Journal of the American Medical Association, 261,* 2543–2545.

Riesenberg, D., & Lundberg, G. D. (1990). The order of authorship: Who's on First? *Journal of the American Medical Association, 264,* 1857.

Schain, R. J., & Freedman, D. X. (1961). Studies of 5-hydroxyindole metabolism in autistic and other mentally retarded children. *Journal of Pediatrics, 58,* 315–321.

Sharp, D. W. (1991). Fraud: The journal's role concerning fraudulent research. *Investigative Radiology, 26*(6), 586–589.

— CHAPTER 11 —————————————————————————

The Institutional Review Board: Ethical Gatekeeper

RICHARD L. COHEN, MD
ALEXANDER J. CIOCCA, JD, MPH

HISTORICAL AND LEGAL BASIS

The Institutional Review Board (IRB) is responsible for the review of Department of Health and Human Services (HHS) (1981, 1983) funded research involving human subjects, and it functions within the framework of federal regulations (45 C.F.R. § 46 *et seq.*). Corresponding regulations and guidelines applicable to the IRB are also promulgated by the Food and Drug Administration (FDA) (21 C.F.R. §§ 50, 56 *et seq.*). These governmental regulations and related federal statutes, however, are actually a reflection of society's moral and ethical views. As such, they strive to maintain an appropriate balance between personal dignity and the right to self-determination on one hand, and the overall societal benefit to be derived from research that involves human subject participation on the other.

An authoritative source of basic ethical principles and guidelines for research involving human subjects is the "Belmont Report," published by the National Commission for the Protection of Human Subjects of Biomedical and Behavioral Research (1978). The Commission members who produced the Belmont Report reviewed the most egregious abuses of human subjects used in biomedical research, including the experiments carried out during the World War II that resulted in the Nuremberg Code as an initial template for the ethical treatment of human subjects. The Belmont Report also acknowledges the Helsinki Declaration of 1964, as revised in 1975, the federal regulations concerning IRBs, and the American Psychological Association Code for Social and Behavioral Research, published in 1973. Using these documents as models, the Belmont Report established basic ethical principles for use in human subject research that include respect for persons, beneficence, and justice. Application of these principles may be summarized by stating that human subject research should respect the individual's right to self-determination in the sense of voluntary participation in research. Furthermore, researchers are obligated to maximize benefits and minimize harms to the subject as well as to apply fundamental fairness in overall subject selections, so that minorities, welfare patients, and other potentially compromised groups of human beings are not manipulated into research participation.

The IRB evaluation of human subject research protocols should always involve these basic ethical principles evolving from the Belmont Report. These principles are covered by federal IRB regulations that require voluntary informed consent, accurate description of risks and benefits for participation, and the equitable selection of subjects. The IRB is further obligated to follow additional considerations that may be contained in the institution's Assurance, which is filed by any institution engaged in HHS-funded research. This may involve more detailed and perhaps restrictive interpretations of federal regulations or ethical principles determined as a matter of institutional prerogative.

For example, unless an exception is applicable, the federal regulations concerning elements of informed consent require that the following information be provided to each subject:

1. Statement of the purpose of the research study and procedures to be followed.
2. Description of reasonably foreseeable risks or discomforts as well as benefits expected from the research.
3. Appropriate alternative procedures or courses of treatment.
4. Description of confidentiality of the records and data involved.
5. Whether any compensation or other medical treatment for research-related injury is available.
6. Statement that no penalty will be incurred by virtue of refusing to participate in the research, or extra benefit obtained for participating.
7. Designated source where more information or clarification may be obtained at the institution.

The IRB may require that additional information be given to subjects when in the IRB's judgment, the information would meaningfully add to the protection of the rights and welfare of subjects. Thus, it is clear that the IRB, functioning as the agent of the institution and under the institution's Assurance to HHS, may create operating guidelines, policies, and procedures to implement locally determined ethical and moral judgments aimed at protecting the rights of human subjects.

INSTITUTIONAL LEGAL AND OPERATIONAL PREROGATIVES

The institution may have other legal, operational, and public/community image objectives that it wishes to maintain and that overlap to some degree with human subject research. For example, institutions that receive HHS funds for research generally are nonprofit and tax-exempt educational corporations, such as universities, colleges, and medical research complexes. The mission of such an organization would be to carry out academic, research, and clinical service functions for public benefit (Kobasic, 1988; Levine, 1986). In return for this public benefit, the federal government, and to varying degrees state and local governments, confer on such organizations tax-exempt status that is implicitly contingent on continuous operation as a public charity. The definition and interpretation of a "public charity" varies among governmental units. Such benefits may include exemption from income taxation, property taxation, and direct public funding for such activities. When human subject research is carried out in university facilities and under its auspices in a tax-exempt environment, then the university has additional (perhaps self-serving to some degree) reasons to ensure that human subject research and the conduct of the researchers themselves are truly consistent with public benefit.

Most universities have guidelines and principles with respect to situations involving conflict of interest or conflict of commitment on behalf of its faculty, staff, and students. These guidelines and principles are, for the most part, general in nature, and they require application many times on a case-by-case basis, similar to the manner in which the basic ethical principles illustrated in the Belmont Report would be applied by any IRB evaluation of human subject research. In 1989, the NIH and ADAMHA combined to publish for comment a more detailed set of conflict of interest guidelines for federally funded researchers (Bick, 1989). These proposed regulations required significant disclosure of potential conflict information by researchers. They appear to take the ethical principles of the Belmont Report one step further, aiming to protect and ensure public confidence in the results obtained thereby. This proposal was withdrawn after much public clamoring that it was too restrictive and detrimental to private- and public-sponsored research, which is then commercialized for societal benefit. Clearly, however, the commercial research results also benefit private profit motives of proprietary research sponsors and the researcher/inventor.

Whether an institution should, particularly through its IRB, be more scrutinizing of human subject research vis-à-vis institutional objectives (e.g., retaining tax-exempt status, maintaining public confidence, and preventing unacceptable conflicts of interest) is an issue that remains open. The positive effects of addressing the issue should be sufficiently significant to prompt heightened awareness and meaningful discussion at an institution. Although it may be said that the IRB is the ethical gatekeeper to human subject research with the minimal difficulty of gate opening set by federal regulations, any additional "spring tension" to the gate may be applied by institutional prerogative. The institution and its researchers and their subjects would all benefit if the IRB was a key part of such action.

SCIENTIFIC MISCONDUCT IN HUMAN SUBJECT RESEARCH MONITORING AND REPORTING

Institutions receiving federal funding from the HHS are required, effective January 1, 1990, to establish a policy and procedure for review and investigation of scientific misconduct allegations. The term *misconduct* includes conduct that seriously deviates from accepted research practices (including federal requirements for protection of human subjects). Fabrication, falsification, and plagiarism are specific cited examples of misconduct. Not included are honest error or honest differences in interpretations or judgments of data. Institutions are required to have in place a process for initial review of a scientific misconduct allegation to determine if it has sufficient substance to warrant further review. This phase is termed an inquiry, whereas a further review is an investigation. Both have specific time periods for reaching conclusions and include basic elements of due process (i.e., notice to the accused and opportunity to respond to the charge in an organized fashion). Findings and recommendations, if any, of the investigative process may be subject to further review by appeal. Notification to the NIH Office of Scientific Integrity (OSI) is required under various circumstances. The OSI may elect to conduct its own investigation (42 C.F.R. § 50.101 *et seq.*).

The federal regulations specifically applicable to human subject research and the IRB likewise require the reporting of regulatory violation or noncompliance by investigators, which may also meet the definition of *scientific misconduct*. However, such reporting does not require a lengthy internal review process to be initiated concurrently as with the misconduct regulations. Rather, the IRB is charged with the responsibility and authority to carry out whatever remedial action is appropriate to protect human research subjects in a summary and timely manner. This may include immediate termination of the research and notification to subjects at risk. The investigative aspect apparently could be carried out by the NIH Office for Protection from Research Risks (OPRR) (45 C.F.R. § 46.108). For the research of products regulated by the FDA, the sponsor or investigator has the responsibility of reporting problems to the FDA, which could also investigate the situation (21 C.F.R. § 56.108).

Reviews of the conduct of the investigator in question could apparently occur by the OSI, OPRR, FDA, and internally by the institution in an overlapping concurrent manner. All would be aimed at protecting the public in some way from alleged deviant research practices. However, the federal agencies may also be interested in recovering funds spent on fraudulent or nonconforming research, and for possibly initiating criminal charges against alleged violators. Institutional interests may be aimed at determining appropriate sanctions against the investigator (if found guilty of misconduct), including possible employment termination, as well as protecting or rehabilitating the public image of the institution and its overwhelming majority of responsible investigators.

Where does this leave the IRB? It is (1) the evaluation and authorization mechanism for beginning the research, (2) the monitor for purposes of continuation, and (3) the whistle-blower and police officer when ethical, regulatory, or scientific misconduct is suspected or apparent. Although all of these roles are part of the IRB job description, most would agree that emphasis and resources are principally expended in the evaluation and authorization area. Some might say that investigation and enforcement areas are the responsibility of other institutional organizational components. It is fair to say that the IRB, through its multidisciplinary membership, has a definite interest in protecting human subjects in research, and therefore, if that requires taking further, even drastic action, it must be done in a responsible timely manner. It is a most delicate task to act fairly on a report that may identify an alleged perpetrator of fraud or misconduct and simultaneously protect research subjects as well as the reputation of the identified investigator. Balancing the rights of each requires institutional support, confidential communication, and cohesiveness so that the IRB may proceed in a proper fashion, and in conjunction with other parts of the institution and applicable federal agencies (Christakes, 1988; Hilgartner, 1990; Wegodsky, 1984).

TYPES OF MISCONDUCT AND FRAUD

Coercion of Subjects

Coercion of subjects to enroll in a particular protocol must be termed misconduct because (1) it may expose subjects to unnecessary or unwarranted risk or expense, (2) it may influence them to relinquish a treatment option that they would otherwise prefer, or (3) it may involve illegal or unethical penalties for not participating in a project.

A common example involves the recruitment of students as research subjects. When this is done under the guise of offering training in the conduct of research whereas the underlying intent is simply to recruit a population of captive subjects, the practice cannot be condoned. Students may especially feel coerced because they believe they will receive poor grades unless they "volunteer." This belief is further reinforced if the students are explicitly informed that they will receive course credit for participating. Very often, inspection of the protocol reveals that the students will actually receive no specific training in research.

Other forms of coercion occur when subjects are (1) led to believe that they will give up some of their rights to treatment (present or future) if they do not enroll in a protocol; (2) offered exorbitant payment (e.g., several hundred dollars for a few hours of time) to participate; (3) not provided with all of the information about alternate forms of treatment currently available; or (4) influenced by extravagant and/or premature claims by the investigator (usually disseminated in the media) about a new agent, device, or procedure. The practice is particularly coercive if the investigator is a nationally prominent person and/or the institution is a prestigious one.

Item 4 may involve yet another level of coercion. The IRB itself may find that it is under pressure to approve a project because some combination of consumers, institutional administrators, and manufacturing interests are convinced by what they have read and viewed in the public media. Whether this pressure is intentional and has been planned by the investigators, or is an unintentional by-product of public interest in a high-profile disease, this still constitutes a form of coercion. As such, it must be dealt with firmly by the IRB.

"Bootlegging" Research

It is not uncommon for a clinical investigator to stretch credibility by performing an elaborate list of laboratory and radiological studies on a group of patients suffering from a poorly understood disease, and then attempting to justify this action as the "gold standard" of practice.

In fact, this may be a technique for avoiding the exigencies of research peer review, the perils of research funding, and the sometimes difficult task of eliciting informed consent from potential subjects.

At the same time, the investigator is amassing a large data pool that may serve as the basis for one or more contributions to the scientific literature (enhancing his or her own career status) and/or potentially valuable intellectual property (enriching his or her own pocketbook).

This practice is not acceptable because it may expose subjects to significantly increased risk (depending on the nature of the studies) and to major increases in the cost of care either directly, or indirectly through third party payors, all without informed consent.

Failure to Inform

During a clinical research project, it is not unusual for new information about the disease, its diagnosis, or treatment to become available. This may emerge from the work of the present project or from the reports of others in the field. In any case, it may be information that might cause some subjects to rethink their decision to participate in the project.

Perhaps other treatments have become available. Perhaps they have been shown to incur lower levels of risk. Perhaps they are more efficacious. Perhaps the agent being studied in the present project has revealed itself to be more toxic in ways that may greatly increase risk. Of consequence, then, the intentional withholding of such information from patients and their families in order to continue the project is reprehensible and constitutes serious scientific misconduct.

Misrepresentation of Coinvestigators

Investigators may list colleagues as participants in a project without the latters' knowledge or permission (and without any serious intent of employing their skills in planning or executing the study). This is usually done to add weight to the investigator's contention that he or she has the resources to complete the project as described, and to deflect possible criticism that the investigator may be deficient in specific areas of scientific background deemed basic to the study.

Aside from the obvious fact that misappropriation of a colleague's name is a breach of academic ethics, this action constitutes research misconduct because it misrepresents the investigator's resources for carrying out the research. It contains an implicit statement that the investigator's credentials cannot stand on their own merit and therefore require the names and reputations of other colleagues. It may also have the effect of placing subjects at higher risk if less experienced investigators are carrying out difficult or new clinical research.

Unauthorized Deception

Occasionally, it may be justifiable to use deception of subjects when doing research. For instance, there may be sufficient reason to allow trained actors to carry out the roles of patients when studying staff observational or interviewing techniques.

This should always be done with prior review and approval by the IRB with appropriate "stop" procedures in the protocol in the event that a specific study episode gets out of control and should always include a terminal debriefing sequence during which the entire process is justified to the subjects.

Unfortunately, the aforementioned is not always the case. For example, the investigator may wish to study the incidence of venereal disease in pregnant teenagers. He advertises in local newspapers that his clinic will offer free prenatal visits, including counseling sessions to adolescents who are pregnant (or who suspect that they are). There is no mention of venereal disease, the purpose of the study, or indeed that it is a study at all.

Yet, if the project is carried out as designed, many young women may have their names placed on a roster of patients with known venereal disease without knowledge that such a roster exists and without control of the use of the information.

The investigator's contention that an adequate number of subjects would never be enrolled in the study without this deception is not an acceptable justification.

Failure to Follow Approved Protocol

Once a protocol and its accompanying consent form(s) have received IRB approval, they should not be modified without further review and approval. Otherwise, investigators who introduce changes are at risk of being charged with misconduct for the following reasons:

1. The modifications may have altered the risk level (e.g., due to the introduction of invasive procedures, exposure to higher levels of radiation, significant increases in the volume of blood being drawn during a brief time span, etc.).
2. Such changes may throw doubt on the worthiness of the project (e.g., if they involve significant changes in design, such as adding or removing a study arm or modifying the format of a drug regimen) therefore causing the IRB to reexamine the risk/benefit equation.
3. The changes may have altered the patient mix (e.g., by changing inclusionary and/or exclusionary criteria) and therefore introduced new questions into the matter of potential risk and benefit.

CONFLICT OF INTEREST

Clearly, an institution may be more restrictive than federal regulations in its requirements for human subject research that is to be conducted under its organizational umbrella. What areas of potential conflict should the IRB review in relation to federal regulations for protection of human subjects, and with respect to directives provided through the institution's Assurance, policies, and own determination of employee conduct? The IRB is both fact finder and judge in this complex scenario.

For example, most if not all universities permit private consulting by faculty to the extent that such activity is not done on university time or with its resources and does not constitute a conflict of interest vis-à-vis the university and the faculty member's university duties. When the faculty member is also conducting human subject research that may involve aspects of the private consulting arrangement, then the question arises as to what type of disclosure is required to adequately inform the human subjects? This, of course, would be a locally determined matter, but the principal issues are the following:

1. Disclosure of the private consulting arrangements and overlap with the particular research project may be important to achieve fully informed consent.
2. Nondisclosure may be interpreted as a bias or influencing factor on the part of the investigator.

3. Nondisclosure may also be viewed as willful concealment and thus as a factor that taints the research and that may result in a loss of public confidence in the institution, the researcher, and the private sponsor and its product.

It is also important to note that most universities have written policies applicable to intellectual property produced by faculty, staff, and students. In many such policies, the university owns the product and the inventor shares to varying degrees in any proceeds that result from the sale, licensing, or other commercialization of the invention. Occasionally, such inventions are sold or licensed to a third party private business in which the researcher or his family holds equity, board positions, or employment arrangements for which compensation is provided. It is even more complicated where the institution may itself hold equity. These arrangements may be made in advance of human subject research being carried out and without notification to subjects. Without advance disclosure of such ties, the potential for perceived conflict of interest or commitment may be heightened to a degree that is disturbing to the public. It seems clear that disclosure is the first element in addressing and preventing these potential problems.

Even after disclosure is provided, how is the IRB to evaluate such disclosures in a "balancing of interests" test, protecting the rights of human subjects while allowing the investigator to carry out his or her research activities?

For example, assume that a faculty member has invented a novel and potentially clinically important product to which he or she holds ownership or royalty rights. The faculty member then discloses this information to the IRB in the desire to conduct further research and development on the product involving human subjects, and with sponsorship by a private company to whom the product has been sold or licensed. How can the IRB approve such human subject research and feel comfortable that the potential private gain for the researcher will not influence his or her conduct in the project? How can the IRB reduce the potential for shortcuts or for the production of less than accurate, misrepresentative, or selective data that could have detrimental effects on the human subjects involved as well as the public if the product is then approved for general use? On the other hand, how can the IRB, particularly at an academic institution, disapprove such research without interfering with the academic freedom of the investigator?

One course of action could be to disapprove such research as unduly compromising the position of participants. This could be done as institutional policy or on a case-by-case basis. Another would be to insist that the study be carried out by investigators who do not share in any potential profits from the success of the product. As another alternative, initial review of the study by peers in the investigator's department could occur prior to IRB review. If approved, some typ^ of additional oversight committee composed of appropriately experienced scientists or physicians could be impaneled thereafter to periodically review the specific research activities as well as the data produced by the investigator. The latter approach would be a middle ground between complete disapproval and no disclosure or monitoring whatsoever. In addition, of course, full disclosure to subjects could be mandated.

Do the scenarios put the IRB and its membership in an untenable position? It is quite possible for this to be the case if the IRB membership for whatever reason would accede to pressure from the investigator in question, who may in fact be a colleague, and/or from institutional administrators desirous of an improved research funding pool, as well as potential commercialization revenues from inventions. Additional reasonable reviews of such scenarios by other organizational components should reduce the potential for unwise decisions. It would seem that a case-by-case determination may be the only way to resolve these problems. Involvement of a case precedent system would be essential to ensure that IRB review of such matters is being done in a fair and consistent manner. This would presumably benefit the subjects, the investigator, the institution, the IRB and all other concerned parties.

Potential IRB Actions in Suspected Cases of Misconduct or Fraud

Because of the credibility usually enjoyed by the IRB, it should be particularly cautious about arriving at premature judgments concerning scientific misconduct. Meticulous attention to the principles of due process is essential. Unsupportable accusations (or inferences) have an impact on both the professional and lay communities. It is unforgivable to tarnish a reputation and perhaps to hamper a bright career with premature or frivolous claims of wrongdoing.

Local practice will determine the specific responsibilities of the IRB to conduct inquiries and to take whatever action it deems warranted based on the findings of such inquiry. However, certain generalities apply in most settings.

Initial Review of Submission and Data Collection

It is possible to anticipate certain types of possible misconduct a priori at the point when the project is submitted for its initial review. As always, it is best to deal with potential misconduct preventively rather than after the fact. Most common among such actions are the following:

Coercive Practices. Is it clear that there will be no penalties invoked if potential subjects (patients, students, controls) refuse to participate? Are subject compensation fees excessive? Are extravagent claims made for untested treatments? Is information about possible alternative treatments withheld or minimized?

Deceptive Practices. Has there been a full description of the nature and purpose of the project? Of the procedures that will be performed? Of the risks attendant to these? Of alternative forms of treatment available? Of confidentiality practices? If deception is deemed an essential aspect of the design, is the justification adequate and has an adequate debriefing been provided so that subjects eventually are fully informed?

Misrepresentation of Faculty. Have procedures been observed that require each investigator to sign the protocol attesting to his or her willingness to participate and to personal knowledge of its contents?

Conflicts of Interest. Has there been disclosure both to the IRB and to potential subjects concerning the costs of the project, how these will be met, and whether or not the investigators have any direct or indirect financial interest in it? Does the project impact or involve overlap with private consulting arrangements with "spin off" or privately held companies, or royalty arrangements in which the investigator may participate?

Informal Unsolicited Reports from Staff, House Officers, and Subjects

Without specific intent, IRBs often come into possession of information about a project from collateral sources. These are usually well-intentioned individuals who perceive that some abuse is being perpetrated by one or more investigators. It is therefore logical that the former should then turn to the official body that has been charged with protecting subjects from such abuse.

Unfortunately, there may also be instances when the whistle-blower may be entertaining a less altruistic agenda. Conflicts and tensions existing between individual faculty members may tempt someone to report malicious gossip as fact or to interpret an innocent act of omission as intentional wrongdoing. It is therefore incumbent on the IRB to *proceed with extreme caution until such reports can be independently substantiated.*

At the same time dismissing such reports out of hand is not advisable. House officers and nursing staff are particularly sensitive to attempts to bootleg research; the hospital pharmacy is a reliable source about requests for experimental drugs that exceed approved levels of sample size for a given protocol; and investigator colleagues often become aware that the "Methods Section" of an experiment is not being carried out as it was originally described.

When reports of such misconduct are received, it is vital to confidentially notify the principal investigator of this at once and to request an interview with the Chair of the IRB. This procedure is an essential aspect of the data collection process. Written minutes of the allegations and discussions at such meetings should be retained. Depending on the gravity of the charges, it may be advisable to have a third party present (preferably another experienced IRB member). At times, the concerns prove to be the result of a misunderstanding and can be quickly resolved. If this is not the case, then the inquiry must be continued to include all relevant data. Notification of other internal and external authorities must be considered in a timely and appropriate manner consistent with institutional policy.

Monitoring and Follow-up Review

It is customary for IRBs to monitor the status of ongoing research in a structured and organized fashion. Federal regulations require this approach, but in any case, it makes eminent sense to do so because many unanticipated risks (and benefits) can arise as the work progresses.

The follow-up activity may take several forms including:

Review of requests for renewal of project and attendant risks.

Review of requests for modifications.

Adverse reaction reports.

Published reports of findings.

Gross discrepancies between descriptions of the project as originally approved and the work as it is later represented should become apparent. A frequent illustration of this has to do with major deviations from approved procedures. In this case, involvement of other appropriate institutional officials and federal agencies in the process should be sought.

Reporting

Federal regulations and institutional policies dictate to whom and under which circumstances information concerning actual or alleged scientific misconduct must be reported. The IRB has authority under federal law to suspend or terminate approval of research if it is not being conducted in accordance with the IRB's requirements or if it proves to be associated with unexpected serious harm to subjects. The IRB is responsible for making a prompt report of the suspension or termination of approval, including reasons therefor, and directing the report to the investigator, appropriate institutional officials, and the NIH Office for Protection from Research Risks (45 C.F.R. § 46.113). The Department of HHS (1989) has authority to require termination or suspension of funding for any research project where an institution has materially failed to comply with federal regulations concerning protection of human subjects. Such action by the Department of HHS may influence future HHS funding applications or proposals by the affected institution and/or investigator (45 C.F.R. § 46.123).

The FDA places the burden for prompt reporting of unanticipated problems on the sponsor and investigator. The FDA also provides sanctions for regulatory noncompliance (21 C.F.R. § 56.120-124). Nonetheless, the IRB could terminate or suspend the study approval and make such a report if the sponsor or investigator fails to do so.

Institutional policy for reporting scientific misconduct must comply with federal law, as noted previously. Although the procedure for carrying out the intent of the policy may vary somewhat among institutions, the responsible institution must comply at a minimum with federally mandated requirements, including timeframes for review and reporting.

The IRB is likely to be the locus of initial reporting for scientific misconduct information about human subject research and the investigator carrying it out. Initiating prompt action to protect the research subjects' rights should be the IRB's first thrust. After this objective has been met, timely and confidential review of the situation should occur with appropriate institutional officials to address the various external reporting requirements that may be applicable. Due consideration should be given to many factors prior to making a report, including without limitation: credibility of the evidence supporting the initial allegations and the investigator's response, the degree of risk, contractual obligations also to notify the sponsor of the research, and the confidential nature of the communications. A diligently prepared, accurate, and appropriately worded report benefits all concerned parties. Although the need for such reporting may occur infrequently, an established and well-understood institutional procedure should nonetheless be available to the IRB for such instances.

SUMMARY

The IRB is a key player in the processes of review, approval, and monitoring for human subject research, and for the detection and confrontation of possible scientific misconduct. Clearly this is a multidimensional program with institutional and federal involvement. As the "public's right and desire to know" has continued to increase, and institutions are under more public scrutiny with respect to the propriety of actions by their investigators, staff, and students, it would appear that the time is right to address these issues in a responsible coordinated fashion. Federal guidelines on such issues may be helpful. However, the institution's own prerogative to establish and maintain adherence to appropriate principles for research may be more important to human research subjects. It will certainly be a major factor in determining public confidence in the institution. Established mechanisms for conflict disclosure and review may help to limit the potential for circumvention, disregard, or the appearance of impropriety concerning basic issues of human research and scientific conduct. The likelihood that flagrant ethical violators will be discovered may increase, whereas potential conflicts for the legitimate investigator who properly discloses should be eased.

The gateway into the research arena is to a large degree opened by the IRB; likewise, the monitoring and removal of unethical entrants is a responsibility to society that the IRB must exercise appropriately.

REFERENCES

Bick, K. (1989). Request for comment on proposed guidelines for policies on conflict of interest (developed by the National Institutes of Health and Alcohol, Drug Abuse, and Mental Health Administration). *NIH Guide for Grants and Contracts, 18,* 1–5.

Christakes, N. A. (1988, March/April). Should IRBs monitor research more strictly?. *IRB: A Review of Human Subjects Research,* Vol. 10, pp. 8–10.

Department of Health and Human Services, Food and Drug Administration. (1981). Title 21 Code of Federal Regulations, Parts 50 and 56.

Department of Health and Human Services, National Institutes of Health, Office for Protection from Research Risks. (1983). Title 45 Code of Federal Regulations, Part 46.

Department of Health and Human Services, National Institutes of Health, Office of Scientific Integrity. (1989). Title 42 Code of Federal Regulations, Part 50.

Hilgartner, S. (1990, Jan./Feb.). Research fraud, misconduct and the IRB. *IRB: A Review of Human Subjects Research,* Vol. 12, pp. 1–4.

Kobasic, D. M. (1988). Institutional Review Boards in the university setting: Review of pharmaceutical testing protocols, informed consent and ethical concerns. *Journal of College and University Law, 15,* 185–216.

Levine, Robert J. (1986). The Institutional Review Board. In *Ethics and regulations of clinical research* (2nd ed., pp. 321–363). Baltimore: Urban and Schwarzenberg, Inc.

National Commission for the Protection of Human Subjects of Biomedical and Behavioral Research. (1978). Belmont Report. Washington, DC: Author.

Wegodsky, H. S. (1984, March/April). Fraud and misrepresentation in research—Whose responsibility? *IRB: A Review of Human Subjects Research,* Vol. 6, pp. 1–5.

— SECTION IV

Epilogue

Future Directions: A Modest Proposal

MICHEL HERSEN, PhD
DAVID J. MILLER, PhD

INTRODUCTION

Scarely a month goes by without a new instance of research fraud in the biomedical and social sciences being reported in the media (e.g., Ear Center, 1990; Pitt Doctor's Writing, 1990; Question of Scientific Fakery, 1989; Two Pitt Researchers, 1990) or professional newsletters and journals (e.g., FDA Challenges, 1988; Fraud Issue, 1989; Shapiro & Charrow, 1985). Although it might be tempting to attribute the seemingly alarmingly high number of new cases to intensified academic pressures in our time or to increased vigilance of the scientific community in the 1980s and 1990s (Garfield, 1990; Institute of Medicine, 1989), a more sobering thought emerges after a careful reading of Broad and Wade's (1982) *Betrayers of the Truth: Fraud and Deceit in the Halls of Science*. Indeed, the names of the prior cases of scientific fraud or misconduct listed by Broad and Wade (e.g., Ptolemy, Galileo, Newton, Bernoulli, Dalton, Mendel, Peary, Millikan) identify and indict a veritable who's who in the history of science. Thus, albeit a "relatively" infrequent phenomenon, scientific fraud has an extremely lengthy history, implicating many famous individuals. Perhaps the potential notoriety associated with important scientific discovery attracts some individuals with an unscrupulous bent to the field. But equally plausible, and also sobering is the thought that most likely science does not attract a substantially greater percentage of unscrupulous individuals than any other professional group (e.g., politicians, theologians, athletes, industrialists, bankers, and stockbrokers).

Because it is predominantly in the past decade that scientists and others have recognized the problem of research fraud in the biomedical and social sciences (Blakely, Poling, & Cross, 1986; Greene, Durch, Horwitz, & Hooper, 1986; Tangney, 1987), it is difficult to determine whether such fakery, plagiarism, and other misdeeds are on the increase. That is, we simply do not have the requisite baseline data to make this kind of an assessment. On the basis of our ensuing analysis of the factors contributing to the problem, we will offer a number of solutions to keep fraudulent activity to a minimum. We do recognize, however, that irrespective of the preventive and curative efforts carried out, undoubtedly a certain percentage of individuals will still transgress. The notion that there is a genetic predisposition to conduct disorder and psychopathy leads to the conclusion that through associative mating the gene will continue to be expressed and the behavioral sequelae will follow. Perhaps for such individuals no preventive strategies will work. On the other hand, those individuals who proceed in a moral and honest fashion may have little need for carrying out preventive measures. But there may be still a third group, who have the proclivity and who will swerve to the side of honesty with carefully designed prevention. Irrespective of the character of the individuals targeted for preventive efforts, the respective pressures that lead to dishonesty in science must be carefully delineated, articulated, and debated in the literature, and probably reversed to effect rational change. The status quo that perhaps has contributed heavily to the problem cannot be tolerated at the individual, institutional, or systems levels.

The reaction to the number of reports of research fraud and other scientific misconduct in the biomedical and social sciences has been considerable. Tangible responses have occurred at both the local and national levels. Locally, individual universities and research centers have started to develop policies to deal with instances of research fraud. Also, some discussion and efforts at prevention have begun to emerge.

Nationally, in the late 1980s the response has been truly spectacular. In 1985 an article published in the *American Psychologist* (Miers, 1985) stated the National Institute of Health's perspectives on misconduct in science, and it was clear that procedures and policies for dealing with such misconduct were under consideration and being developed. In 1989 the American Psychological Association established a special task force to consider ethical issues related to publication in their numerous journals (Fraud Issue, 1989). As a consequence, beginning in 1990 in the first issue of each APA journal a short policy statement concerning ethics appeared. Also, in 1989 the American Psychological Association announced (Science Directorate, 1989) the appointment of a Research Ethics Officer, serving "as staff liaison to the APA's Committee on Animal Research and Ethics (CARE) and Committee for the Protection of Human Participants in Research (CPHPR). She will also work in the area of fraud and misconduct, representing the interests of research psychologists both in legislative and public education arenas" (p. 51).

Effective July 1, 1990, the National Institutes of Health and the Alcohol, Drug Abuse, and Mental Health Administration adopted a policy that all institutional training grant applications were to include both informal and formal methods related to the "instructions about the responsible conduct of research (NIH, 1990)." This measure obviously, and for good reasons, was directed to the more junior researchers emerging in the field—a group at higher risk for the commission of ethical misconduct.

In 1989 the Institute of Medicine published its lengthy report entitled: *The Responsible Conduct of Research in the Health Sciences.* This report was formulated by individuals representing Councils of the National Academy of Sciences, the National Academy of Engineering, and the Institute of Medicine. The final report consisted of (1) a summary statement that considered the purpose of the study, the assumptions and findings, and the recommendations; (2) history of the issues; (3) key issues tackled in the workshop; (4) analysis of the findings; and (5) recommendations for (a) the National Institutes of Health, (b) universities and other research centers, and (c) professional and scientific organizations and journals. In addition, numerous appendices dealing with a whole host of ethical issues were included.

Listed below are summaries of the recommendations from the Institute of Medicine Report (1989) for universities and other research centers:

> Universities, medical schools, and other research organizations should adopt guidelines to clarify the expectations of each institution about the professional standards to be observed by investigators in the conduct of research. (p. 29)

> Universities should provide formal instruction in good research practices. This instruction should not be limited to formal courses but should be incorporated into various places in the undergraduate and graduate curricula for all science students. (p. 30)

> Universities should designate one or more administrative officers or faculty members to promote responsible research practices within the institution. The institution should also provide mediation and counseling services for faculty, staff, and students who wish to express concerns about professionally questionable training or research practices. (p. 31)

> Universities and other research institutions should strengthen the integrity and quality of research by modifying incentives and academic guidelines in order to reduce the pressure for excessive publication. (p. 31)

> Academic departments and research units should monitor the supervisory and training practices of their faculty and research staff to ensure that adequate oversight is provided for young scientists. (p. 33)

> Academic departments and research units should adopt authorship policies to improve the publication practices of their faculty, staff, and students. (p. 34)

In addition to the reaction that has taken place in academic circles, the government (Walsh, 1990), through Congress, has taken an interest in research fraud and other scientific misconduct, especially since a good number of fraudulent incidents were associated with research grants funded by federal agencies. Under the Chairmanship of Repre-

sentative Ted Weiss (D-NY), the Human Resources and Intergovernmental Relations Subcommittee conducted a 3-year study of
a total of 10 cases of scientific misconduct at Harvard University,
University of Florida, University of Pittsburgh, University of California at San Diego, and Yeshiva University (Committee on Government
Operations, 1990). In each instance the alleged misconduct was
perpetrated during the course of grant work funded by one of the
Public Health Service Agencies. In general, the report is highly
critical of the universities where such transgressions have occurred,
pointing to the universities' "reluctance" to find their own faculty
guilty. The investigative efforts of the universities is considered to be
"inadequate," and evidence is cited showing that the "whistle-blowers" often become the targets of retaliation. However, the final report
certainly does not unanimously reflect all of the committee members'
positions. Indeed, appearing at the conclusion of the report are dis-
senting views that question (1) the "factual accuracy" of the data
reported, (2) the recommendations, and (3) "the questionable injection of Congress into a bitterly ongoing legal dispute."

We obviously do not have sufficient data available to make judgments on the factual accuracy of the final report. But we certainly do
have concerns about these important scientific, legal, ethical, and
moral issues becoming sensationalized and perhaps becoming grist for
political advancement and gain. That, in our opinion, should not be
the object of the exercise. Indeed, it truly detracts from the imperative
of carefully considering the issues and looking for remediation. We
also would argue that, although the reports of the Institute of Medicine (1989) and the Committee on Government Operations (1990) have
elucidated a number of the critical issues, we are not convinced that
sufficient attention has been accorded to what we believe is the *heart
of the problem: the commercialism of academia and its attendant
issues.* Thus, in the remainder of this chapter we will direct our
attention to such issues, including academia as big business, "publish
or perish," publish *positive* results or perish," the fallout of academic
enterpreneurship, the lack of careful mentorship, and the anti-intellectual climate that is pervading the academic atmosphere.

ACADEMIA AS BIG BUSINESS

There was a time, in the "ivory tower" days of academia when knowledge was treasured for its intrinsic value, and the Renaissance individual, who had a comprehensive view of the issues, was considered to be the model. Although publication and the securing of grant monies were an element of the academes' existence, equally important were their teaching abilities and, in the medical arena, their clinical acumen. Although the tripartite role of academicians is still in place, the pendulum has swung in favor of the research endeavor. Indeed, there is no doubt that when promotion is at question, much greater weight is given to the candidates' research contributions than to their teaching, community service, or clinical work with patients. Along with the emphasis on research and successful grant procurement, there has been inevitable specialization resulting from research aimed to fulfill the priorities of the national funding agencies. Thus, investigators, at times, if they choose to "play the game according to the implicit rules," must alter their research directions in line with the external incentives, but not necessarily as a consequence of the data that have been accrued. Admittedly, the identification and selection of priorities has its benefits in the health field, but on the other hand it potentially stifles creativity in regimenting the scientist's inquisitive bent.

One of the limitations of the current system is the highly commercialized approach to research that has evolved during the past 20 years, and in particular within the past decade (see Agnew, 1990; Johnston, 1990). Unfortunately, a market mentality to research has emerged, with academic departments in medical schools often being guided by fiscal considerations rather than academic ones. In a good number of medical schools astronomically large budgets have appeared over time for some departments. Such budgets are inflated with the so-called soft monies adduced via the overhead paid through grants secured from federal funding agencies. In the more active and renowned research institutions the press to maintain and increase these alarmingly high budgets is ever present. Indeed, universities that attract the most grant monies are also obviously the ones that recruit competitive young researchers who wish to "play the research funding game." However, the inevitable fallout is that the financial prize often assumes greater import than the project (i.e., carrying out the research with precision, dedication, and a thirst for new knowledge) for which that prize was originally awarded.

In considering this situation it would be easy to pinpoint the blame on university administrators, department chairpeople, the funding agencies, or the aggressive young researchers who have decided to compete in the arena. To do so, however, would be akin to presenting a specious argument in a court of law, because each element in this game has contributed equally to the problem and at present is moving in circular fashion, unable to extricate itself from the whirlpool of activity. It is equally important, however, to consider dispassionately the consequences of the prolific commercialization of academia. Therefore, in the succeeding sections we will specifically evaluate the elements that directly or indirectly are related to academic commercialism.

PUBLISH OR PERISH

The credo of publishing or perishing in academia certainly is not a 20-century innovation; it literally has been with us for centuries. Indeed, success in the scientific arena has always been measured, to one extent or another, by the scientist's literary productivity, presumably describing innovation, change, criticism, or confirmation. Innovation and change, of course, have always attracted the most attention and have brought about the greatest notoriety for the particular scientist.

In the first half of this century, before publication activity was linked to competing for grant funding, the author's publication record served as an index to determine promotion up the academic ladder, from instructor or assistant professor to the highest possible level (i.e., tenured full professor). In determining whether a promotion was merited, a number of departments had precise criteria for the various academic levels, in some instances assigning weights to number of articles, the quality of the journal in which they were published, and the order of authors in multiauthored papers. However, in most academic departments such precision was, and still is, not the case. To the contrary, a multitude of factors appear to contribute to a positive decision to promote, including the personality features of the candidates and their ability to teach and perform clinical services. However, for those who have attended departmental promotion meetings, and medical school and graduate school promotion committees, there is strong element of "different strokes for different folks." The scientific precision and objectivity, ostensibly characteristic of the research work of such committee members, is usually absent from these deliberations, where emotion at times outranks reasonable choice. However, no matter how much the nonpublication factors are underscored, there remains the tendency to count number of publications and to report whether that number is less, equal to, or more than others who have achieved the academic rank in question. Quality of the work reported is taken into account, but total number of papers published and accepted into peer-reviewed journals always appears in the subcommittee chairperson's report. Caveat emptor! At these meetings members do hear the frequently quoted statement, "There are Nobel Prize winners who have achieved the ultimate honor with less than a dozen publications." But how often are we dealing with Nobel Prize winners or such potential laureates in our committee deliberations?

A strategy for dealing with the publish or perish dilemma has been proposed in the Institute of Medicine Report (1989). This Report made the point, "Not only does the pressure to publish lead to the practices of repetitive publication, trivial work, and loose authorship, but it may also tempt researchers to engage in serious misconduct to achieve publishable results" (p. 32). Thus:

One way of dealing with the deleterious effects of excessive publication pressure is to allow only a limited number of publications to be considered for academic appointment, promotion, or funding. Harvard Medical School, which at one time required a researcher to have a minimum number of publications to be considered for appointment as assistant professor on the basic science faculty, now has guidelines suggesting maximum numbers of publications to be considered for promotion or appointment to each faculty level: 5 for assistant professor, 7 for associate professor, and 10 for full professor. . . .

For such a scheme to have the desired effect of reversing the trend toward greater numbers of publications, it will be essential that the candidate submit a list of only the maximum number of publications allowed (presumably those considered the best) without mentioning others. Only in this way can the emphasis on numbers be changed. (p. 32)

Whether this scheme can be effective is at present a matter for conjecture and in the future a matter for empirical study. However, we would question whether the Harvard proposal indeed represents the most realistic approach unless adopted universally, and whether it does have the potential to stifle positive creativity and innovation in those whose ethics are above reproach. Furthermore, simply decreasing the number of publications required for promotion or obtaining grants is not at all an insurance against fraudulent intent. Indeed, it might even lead those with fraudulent intent to transgress with greater care, making detection yet more difficult at first.

PUBLISH POSITIVE RESULTS OR PERISH

The issue of publishing positive results or perishing has received inadequate attention in the literature and it may be a significant contributor to the perpetration of research fraud and the perse-veration of erroneous data and conclusions in the literature (cf. Chalmers, 1990; Chalmers, Frank, & Reitman, 1990; Friedman, 1990; Garfield & Welljams-Dorof, 1990; Pfeifer & Snodgrass, 1990; Weisse, 1986). Weisse (1986) has stated the problem succinctly:

> I have often been struck by the predominance of investigators with positive findings, with the naysayers in a distinct minority. On a personal level our studies that challenged some previously reported data or beliefs have always had the most trouble getting published. Particularly galling about such rejections is the fact that those investiga-tions were frequently our most difficult, tedious, and meticulously performed. It had seemed, at times, that the only way to get ahead is to be a perpetual yes-man. (p. 23)

Following his concerns about the predominant interest of editors to publish the work of "yea-sayers," Weisse, a professor of medicine, surveyed all 208 original articles published in the *New England Journal of Medicine* in 1984, the first 100 papers published in the *Annals of Internal Medicine* in 1984, and the first 100 papers published in the *Annals of Surgery* in 1984. Each of these articles was categorized in terms of its conclusions: negative, neutral, or positive. For the *New England Journal of Medicine,* 10% were negative, 10% were neutral, and 80% were positive. For the *Annals of Internal Medicine,* 1% were negative, 10% were neutral, and 89% were positive. For the *Annals of Surgery,* 3% were negative, 6% were neutral, and 91% were positive. In a similar analysis of 100 papers selected at random that were presented in 1984 at the meeting of the American Federation for Clinical Research, 2% were negative, 3% were neutral, and 95% were positive.

The percentages across the three independent journals and the convention presentations are remarkably similar, obviously reflecting the bias of the editors and the selection committee of the American Federation for Clinical Research. However, considering Weisse's opening sentence of his paper ("Harvard's C. Sidney Burwell once said that half of what we teach our medical students will, in time be shown to be wrong but that unfortunately, we do not know which half" [p. 23]), the percentages reported have ominous implications for the accumulation over time of erroneous information that is passed on to our students and colleagues. Although a formal analysis, such as Weisse's has not been carried out in the behavioral sciences, there is no reason to expect a different outcome, given our knowledge of editorial practice.

In his final analysis of the issues, Weisse reexamined the 208 articles from the *New England Journal of Medicine* and found 37 that actually considered prior research and current clinical practice strategies. It is of particular interest that 18 confirmed the earlier work, 9 proved to be inconclusive, *but 10 clearly questioned conclusions of the initial work.* Although not quite the 50% argued by Harvard's C. Sidney Burrell, it seems that more than 25% of the material published is subject to empirical challenge. Moreover, if such studies were to be encouraged by editorial policy, there is no doubt that a greater number would be conducted, perhaps then approaching the 50% figure cited by Burrell.

Irrespective of Weisse's (1986) fascinating findings, the current tendency of journal editors to favor positive reports to the exclusion of disconfirmatory ones places additional pressures on investigators. For those with fraudulent bents, this added ingredient may be sufficient to bring about transgression. Thus, not only must they publish to advance, but they must, in at least 90% of instances, publish positive findings. Unfortunately, these circumstances may even influence generally ethical investigators to cut corners and wander into the grayer areas of scientific misconduct. Chalmers (1990), in the *Journal of the American Medical Association,* has examined one of their grayer areas (i.e., underreporting research) and has actually labeled it as "scientific misconduct." In underreporting research the investigator either decides not to publish nonconfirmatory data altogether *or only reports portions of the research that substantiate the experimental or clinical hypotheses.* Throughout his paper Chalmers details examples of such underreporting and the negative consequences for patients. He argues:

> Selective underreporting of research is almost certainly more widespread and more likely to have adverse consequences for patients than the publication of deliberately falsified data. At least there is an accepted mechanism—attempted replication of reported investigations—for reducing the likelihood of being misled by false inferences based on contrived but fully published reports. No such protective mechanisms currently exists with respect to the apparently systematic tendency to underreport certain kinds of valid research findings. (p. 1405)

ACADEMIC ENTREPRENEURSHIP

Researchers in the academic environment have a long history of supplementing their university salaries by engaging in a wide variety of related activities. The list is quite long and includes seeing clinical patients on a fee-for-service basis during the course of the "research day," consulting with other agencies during regular working hours, editing and writing books, presenting talks in other universities for honoraria, developing patented items that have a high likelihood for commercial success, and editing journals for a yearly stipend and, at times, also for a percentage of the royalties. These activities constitute academic entrepreneurship. The process of "double-dipping" (i.e., being reimbursed for a second activity while on university time) is a rarely challenged staple of the academic scene. In many medical schools the practice is highly reinforced, in that it is given both official sanction and tacit approval. Many university officials appear relieved that outside agencies and businesses are willing to rectify to some extent the discrepancies between salaries that are attained in the commercial world and academia. Furthermore, universities are proud of the products of academic entrepreneurship because they reflect well on the industry of their faculty.

As a corollary, the more successful and renowned the academe is, the more likely he or she will be able to generate extra income-producing activities. Thus, not only does engaging in the "publish or perish" and grant procurement games lead to academic advancement, it obviously has a number of very positive financial concomitants. However, parenthetically we should set the record straight by pointing out that according to the typical standards of big business, the prizes attained by academic entrepreneurs are woefully small. Irrespective of the size of the prize, the individual who engages in academic entrepreneurship is frequently placed in the difficult position of "being beholden to two masters." And in certain circumstances where this happens (but not in the vast majority of cases), such conflict of interest may lead the individual to make conclusions or "bend the data" in a manner inconsistent with scientific veracity.

The most flagrant examples of the aforementioned are those scientists (MD and PhD) who work for or consult with the Tobacco Institute and repeatedly argue against the established link between cigarette smoking and lung cancer. Certainly in these instances the financial rewards offered by the Tobacco Institute color the manner in which these individuals interpret the extant data adduced in favor of the smoking–lung cancer link.

The problems of serving two masters tend, however, to be a bit more subtle than in the cases of the scientists hired by the Tobacco Institute. In our estimation, the most difficult issue in terms of research misconduct involves investigators who are paid by the large pharmaceutical conglomerates to evaluate their new drugs (or older drugs with newer applications). For a variety of reasons these investigators have placed themselves at the highest possible degree of risk with respect to conflict of interest (cf. Cantekin, McGuire, & Potter, 1990; Ear Center, 1990; Input Sought, 1989; Two Pitt Researchers, 1990). Although drug companies may not offer direct payments, they will (1) provide investigators with ample research funding, (2) pay for investigators to report their findings at international conventions (e.g., London, Paris, Geneva, Tokyo, Hong Kong, Australia), (3) provide opportunities for large lecture fees on the national and international circuits. Moreover, obtaining such grant funding, once again enhances the investigator's reputation at the home university. Although the drug companies are prepared to accept whatever results may be adduced by independent experimenters who test their products, the literature on "experimenter bias" elucidates the many factors that can influence both the administration of research and interpretation of findings, even with subhuman species (Rosenthal, 1966). As earlier pointed out by Hersen (1980):

> It may be a truism that any scientist . . . is bound by professional integrity to report his results in an honest and unbiased fashion. However, there are ample data showing that behavioral scientists may be unaware of how their biases are affecting, in subtle fashion, the outcome of their experimenter (cf. Rosenthal, 1966). Rosenthal (1966) clearly shows that in both animal and human research, communication of the experimental hypotheses to the research assistants can result in data favorable to that hypothesis. (p. 58)

Recent examples reported in the press of drug investigators' conflicts of interest highlight the problem of being an unbiased scientist when the drug company is the funding source. As astutely noted by Chalmers (1990), "It is surprising that investigators continue to collaborate in commercially organized research without ensuring that the results of research will be analyzed and reported by people who have no commercial vested interest in selective underreporting" (p. 1407). Once again, caveat emptor!

LACK OF CAREFUL MENTORSHIP

For the most part, recent cases of research fraud (e.g., Norman, 1986) and the vast majority of those transgressions that occurred in the 1970s and early 1980s (see Broad & Wade, 1982) have involved investigators who have been under 40 years of age. These individuals were all junior, in that they were either postdoctoral fellows, assistant professors, or associate professors (see Altman & Melcher, 1983). When the case histories detailed in Broad and Wade are examined carefully, a question arises as to how meticulously and directly these individuals were supervised. It will be recalled that as one of its major recommendations to universities and other research centers, the Institute of Medicine Report (1989) underscores the importance of "adequate oversight . . . for young scientists." In the larger research laboratories and major departments in medical schools such careful oversight has, at times, been given short shrift.

Related to our previous discussion in the section on the academic entrepreneur are those cases of very successful senior researchers who, through their grantsmanship efforts, are able to receive multimillion dollar grants that can provide salary support for many young investigators. Not only do these younger investigators carry out the dictates of the major thrust of the research for the principal investigators (i.e., the senior mentors), but through their resourcefulness they also are able to develop offshoots of the work, thus yielding their own imprints. Unfortunately, in some instances the complexity of the projects, the sheer numbers of people employed in the grant work, and all of the attendant administrative responsibilities faced by the senior researcher (i.e., the principal investigator/mentor) are so overwhelming that careful supervision becomes a secondary concern. Either mentorship is carried out in cavalier fashion, or it is relegated to another faculty person on the research team. When the principal investigator is working on several projects of considerable magnitude, it further compounds the problem. This is frequently the case because, in the competitive world of funding, the "rich get more grants" and the "poor work for those who have grants."

Other instances of inadequate mentorship have been observed by the senior author (MH) of this chapter during the course of his role as a committee member of a medical school promotions committee. On a number of occasions, while serving on such a committee, he has had the opportunity to interview a departmental chairperson about a given candidate being considered for promotion. Remarkably, at times the chair was not always able to make a good case for promotion because of not being "fully familiar with the candidate's activities." Questions about such candidates were referred by the chair to "division supervisors." Admittedly, in large medical school departments, where full-time faculty can exceed 300, the numbers of faculty to be tracked by a chairperson can be staggering. But the sheer lack of knowledge by department chairs in some of these promotion committee interviews is reminiscent of those Roman rulers who had limited knowledge of the activities of their generals and legions in the remote outposts of the

Empire. Just as in the case of the Empire when it expanded too rapidly, inadequate knowledge of the specific activities of the faculty has led to the downfall of some very senior investigators (cf. Altman & Melcher, 1983).

THE ANTI-INTELLECTUAL CLIMATE

The anti-intellectual climate seen in some segments of academia can be traced to the increasing commercialism of the research enterprise and academic entrepreneurship. Although prevalent throughout all of academia, the most striking examples are found in medical schools, where there are very large budgets for given departments. The most flagrant instances, reflective of the anti-intellectual climate, concern grant funding. Here, the heavy emphasis is on securing the grant, with much less concern for what the investigators are studying or what they may ultimately discover as a result of their labors. Comments such as "How much did you get from NIH?" or "How much was the overhead on the grant?" or "How high was your priority score?" are frequently heard on receipt of grants. These are the wrong questions; at best, they should only be secondary or tertiary. The real questions to ask are "What are you planning to study?" "What do you hope to achieve?" "What did you discover in your initial grant application?" "What do your results contribute to the understanding of the illness?" "What strategies do you plan to use now for the 30% who do not get better with Drug X?"

Again, we must stress that because promotion up the academic ladder now is tied in with grant funding, the press on young investigators is to produce and be successful at the national level for funding. The ultimate pressure, then, is to bring in money to the department. Thus, discovery of new information may only be a means to an end rather than an end in itself. Unfortunately, senior mentors as well have become caught up in the proverbial game, reinforcing their students for financial success (i.e., securing large grants) rather than for scientific discovery. Of course, this situation is not a universal feature of medical academia, but it is sufficiently pervasive to warrant concern. The young investigator more interested in glory than scientific fact is especially vulnerable to this system.

RECOMMENDATIONS

The Institute of Medicine Report (1989) has made some excellent recommendations, and we applaud these initial efforts to prevent further occurrences of scientific misconduct in the biomedical and behavioral fields. However, consistent with our analysis of the issues, we would like to add to their list of recommendations. Also, we would like to underscore, in more general terms, the importance of changing the commercial climate that has pervaded our academic environment.

First, we offer the following recommendations:

1. Promotion committees should look at the candidates' work more carefully and determine whether a contribution to the field has been made. Here, innovation, scholarliness, completeness, and thorough grasp of the issues should supersede sheer number of papers published. But, we do not believe the restrictive numerical criteria set by Harvard University will work or that they are necessary.

2. Journal editors should encourage publication of carefully designed and executed studies that refute existing notions in the field. The bias against negative results should be reversed.

3. Promotion to higher ranks should not be unduly influenced by the candidate's grant procurement abilities. Many important discoveries in the biomedical and behavioral science fields have resulted from nonfunded projects. Indeed, the most innovative work does not always get funded.

4. Chairpeople, division leaders, mentors, and senior researchers should be more nurturing of their students and much less concerned whether they will, in time, secure independent funding. The emphasis should be on scientific discovery.

5. Investigators funded by commercial enterprises to evaluate their products should submit research findings to colleagues in the field for independent review, thus being proactive with respect to very possible experimenter bias. Better yet, however, is to avoid the temptation of biasing results, by obtaining grant funding from governmental agencies that "do not have an axe to

grind'' for a specified drug or device. This recommendation certainly augurs better for scientific veracity.

Second, and of considerably greater impact than our specific recommendations, the governmental agencies in power, the administrators in academia, the leading researchers in the field, and the mentors of our more junior faculty must engender in these individuals the thirst for new knowledge and the excitement of discovery. However, in so doing they must repeatedly underline and underscore that there are no shortcuts in science. For the most part, discovery is slow, plodding, painstaking, with the road to ultimate success paved with numerous stumbling blocks, dead ends, and wrong turns. A career in research is not appropriate for those individuals who are impatient and who expect immediate gratification. In this case it is better to be the turtle than the hare.

REFERENCES

Agnew, B. (1990). Delicate conditions: Writing rules for conflict of interest. *The Journal of NIH Research, 2,* 24–27.
Altman, L., & Melcher, L. (1983). Fraud in science. *British Medical Journal, 286,* 2003–2006.
Blakely, E., Poling, A., & Cross, J. (1986). Fraud, fakery, and fudging: Behavior analysis and bad science. In A. Poling and R. W. Fuqua (Eds.), *Research methods in applied behavior analysis* (pp. 313–330). New York: Plenum Press.
Broad, W., & Wade, N. (1982). *Betrayers of the truth.* New York: Simon & Schuster, Inc.
Cantekin, E. I., McGuire, T. W., & Potter, R. L. (1990). Biomedical information, peer review, and conflict of interest as they influence public health. *Journal of the American Medical Association, 263,* 1427–1430.
Chalmers, I. (1990). Underreporting research is scientific misconduct. *Journal of the American Medical Association, 263,* 1405–1408.
Chalmers, T. C., Frank, C. S., & Reitman, D. (1990). Minimizing the three stages of publication bias. *Journal of the American Medical Association, 263,* 1392–1395.
Ear center under federal scrutiny. (1990, Dec. 14). *The Pittsburgh Press,* p. D7.

FDA challenges author of 1986 Alzheimer's study. (1988). *APA Monitor, 19,* 4.

Fraud issue prompts new look at ethics. (1989). *APA Monitor, 20,* 10.

Friedman, P. J. (1990). Correcting the literature following fraudulent publication. *Journal of the American Medical Association, 263,* 1416–1419.

Garfield, E. (1990). The impact of fraudulent research: A citation perspective on the Breuning case. *Current Contents, 12,* 3–4.

Garfield, E., & Welljams-Dorof, A. (1990). The impact of fraudulent research on the scientific literature. *Journal of the American Medical Association, 263,* 1424–1426.

Greene, P. J., Durch, J. S., Horwitz, W., & Hooper, V. S. (1986). Institutional policies for responding to allegations of research fraud. *IRB: A Review of Human Subjects Research, 8,* 1–11.

Hersen, M. (1980). Empirical methods in the behavior disorders. In A. E. Kazdin, A. S.

Bellack, & M. Hersen (Eds.), *New perspectives in abnormal psychology* (pp. 55–80). New York: Oxford University Press.

Input sought on conflict of interest rules. (1989, Dec. 7). *University of Pittsburgh Times,* p. 5.

Institute of Medicine. (1989). Report of a study: *The responsible conduct of research in the health sciences.* Washington, DC: National Academy Press.

Johnston, J. (1990). Universities fire back at misconduct charge. *The Journal of NIH Research, 2,* 29–30.

Miers, M. L. (1985). Current NIH perspectives on misconduct in science. *American Psychologist, 40,* 831–835.

Norman, C. (1986). Senator blasts administration's reinterpretation of ABM Treaty. *Science, 234,* 1489.

Pfeifer, M. P., & Snodgrass, G. L. (1990). The continued use of retracted, invalid scientific literature. *Journal of the American Medical Association, 263,* 1420–1423.

Pitt doctor's writing checked for plagiarism. (1990, March 9). *Pittsburgh Post Gazette.*

Question of scientific fakery is raised in inquiry. (1989, July 12). *The New York Times.*

Rosenthal, R. (1966). *Experimenter effects in behavioral research.* New York: Appleton-Century-Crofts.

Science directorate ethics officer named. (1989). *APA Monitor, 20,* 51.

Shapiro, M. F., & Charrow, R. P. (1985). Special report: Scientific misconduct in investigational drug trials. *New England Journal of Medicine, 312,* 731–738.

Tangney, J. P. (1987, August). *Factors inhibiting self-correction in science.*

Paper presented at the 95th Annual Convention of the American Psychological Association, New York.

Two Pitt researchers accused of misconduct. (1990, Sept. 10). *The Pittsburgh Press.*

Walsh, J. (1990). John Dingell: Demanding humility and fair play from scientists. *The Journal of NIH Research, 2,* 39–43.

Weisse, A. B. (1986). Say it isn't no: Positive thinking and the publication of medical research. *Hospital Practice, March,* 23–25.

Author Index

Subject Index